Keto Diet & Anti-Inflammatory Diet For Beginners 2 in 1

Keto Diet For Beginners

Table of Contents

Anti-Inflammatory Diet For Beginners

Table of Contents

INTRODUCTION

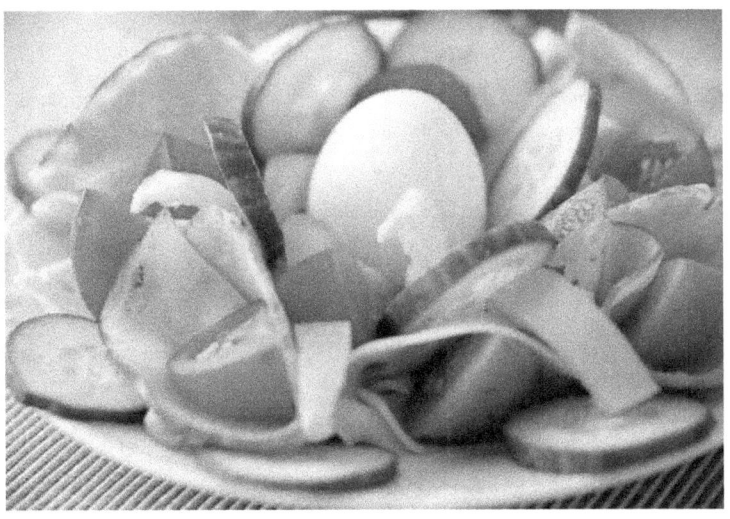

A keto diet is well known for being a low carb diet, where the body produces ketones in the liver to be used as energy. It's referred to as many different names ketogenic diet, low carb diet, low carb high fat (LCHF), etc.

When you eat something high in carbs, your body will produce glucose and insulin.

Glucose is the easiest molecule for your body to convert and use as energy so that it will be chosen over any other energy source.

Insulin is produced to process the glucose in your bloodstream by taking it around the body.

Since the glucose is being used as a primary energy, your fats are not needed and are therefore stored. Typically on a normal, higher carbohydrate diet, the body will use glucose as the main form of energy. By lowering the intake of carbs, the body is induced into a state known as ketosis.

Ketosis is a natural process the body initiates to help us survive when food intake is low. During this state, we produce ketones, which are produced from the breakdown of fats in the liver.

The end goal of a properly maintained keto diet is to force your body into this metabolic state. We don't do this through starvation of calories but starvation of carbohydrates. Reading this Guide will enlight you on the keto diet, stay cool!!

UNDERSTANDING KETOSIS AND KETONES

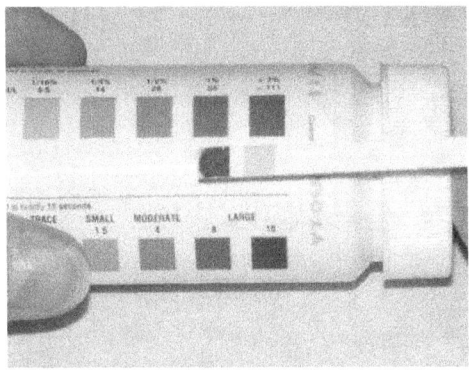

Ketogenic diets are basically designed to induce a state of ketosis in the body. When the amount of glucose in the body becomes too low, the body switches to fat as an alternative source of energy.

The body has two primary fuel sources which are:

Fat deposits are stored in the form of triglycerides. They are normally broken down into long-chain fatty acids and glycerol. Stripping off the glycerol from the triglyceride molecule allows for the release of the three free fatty acid (FFA) molecules into the bloodstream to be used as energy.

The glycerol molecule goes into the liver where three molecules of it combine to form one glucose molecule. Therefore, as your body burns fat, it also produces glucose as a by-product. This glucose can be used to fuel parts of the brain as well as other parts of the body that cannot run on FFA.

However, while glucose can travel through the bloodstream on its own, cholesterol and triglycerides need a carrier to move around in the bloodstream. Cholesterol and triglycerides are packaged in a carrier called low-density lipoprotein, or LDL. Thus, the larger the LDL particle, the more triglycerides it contains.

The overall process of burning fat deposits for energy produces carbon dioxide, water, and compounds called ketones.

Ketones are produced by the liver from free fatty acids. There are composed of 2 groups of atoms linked together by a carbonyl functional group.

The body has no capability to store ketones and therefore they must be either used or excreted. The body excrete them either through the breath as acetone or through the urine as acetoacetate.

Ketones can be used by body cells as a source of energy. Also, the brain can make use of ketones in generating about 70-75% of its energy requirement.

Like alcohol, ketones take priority as a fuel source over carbohydrates. This implies that when they are high in the bloodstream, they must be burned first before glucose can be used as a fuel.

What Causes Ketosis

When you start eating less amounts of carbohydrates, your body gets smaller supply of glucose to use as energy compared to before.

The decrease in the amount of consumed carbohydrates and the subsequent reduction in the amount of available glucose, slowly forces the body to move into the state of ketosis. Thus, the body goes into a state of ketosis when there is not enough amount of glucose available to the body cells.

Starvation Induced Ketosis

Fasting and starvation states usually involve reduced or no intake of food that the body can digest and convert into glucose. While starvation is involuntary, fasting is a more conscious choice you make to intentionally not eat.

However, the body enters into a "starvation mode" whenever you are sleeping, when you skip a meal or when you intentionally go on a fast. The lack of food intake results in a reduction in blood glucose levels. As a result, the body starts to break down it glycogen (stored glucose) stores for energy.

The glycogen is converted back into glucose and used as energy by the body. In this state, the body also starts to burn its stored fats. Thus, the production of ketone bodies (ketogenesis) is induced by a lack of available glucose.

Any time the amount of ketones in the blood outnumber the molecules of glucose, the body cells will start making use of the ketones as their source of energy.

HOW DOES THE KETO DIET WORK

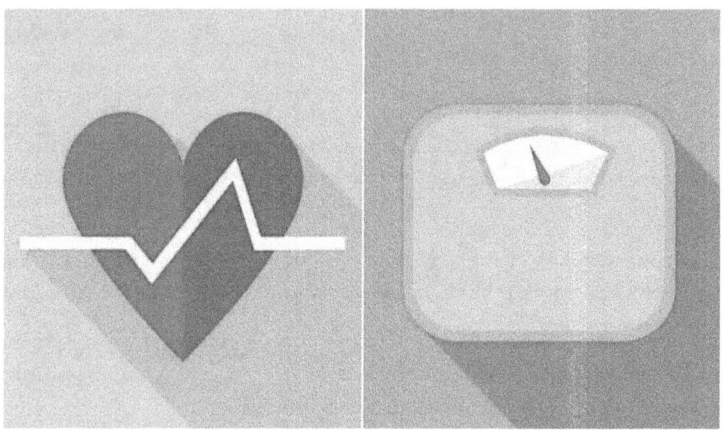

When you eat a diet rich in carbohydrates, your body converts those carbs into glucose (blood sugar). Since carbohydrates are turned into sugar, your blood sugar levels rise.

When blood sugar levels rise, it signals your body to create insulin, which carries glucose to your cells to be used for energy.

Glucose is the preferred energy source of your body. As long as you keep eating carbohydrates, your body will keep turning it into sugar, thereby burning that sugar for energy. In other words, when glucose is present, your body will refuse to burn off its fat stores.

Since carbs are your body's preferred energy source, the only way to start burning fat is by removing carbs.

Cutting carbs depletes your glycogen stores (stored glucose). And with no glucose available for energy, your body has no choice but to start burning its fat stores. Your body starts converting fatty acids into ketones, a metabolic state known as ketosis, and the basis of a ketogenic diet.

What Are Ketones?

In ketosis, your liver converts fatty acids into ketone bodies or ketones. These byproducts become your body's new energy source. When you increase your fat intake, your body responds by becoming "keto-adaptive," or more efficient at burning fat.

Ketosis is a natural survival function of your body. It helps your body function on stored body fat when food is not readily available. Similarly, the keto diet focuses on "starving" your body of carbohydrates, transforming your body into a fat-burning state and supplementing with optimal nutrition.

The three main ketone bodies that your metabolism produces are: Acetoacetate

(AcAc)

Beta-hydroxybutyric acid (BHB) Acetone

The Difference Between Keto, Low-Carb, and Atkins

Too often, the keto diet gets lumped in with other low-carbohydrate diets, like the Atkins Diet. There are a few key differences between them.

Difference In Carbohydrate Intake

The main difference between keto and low-carb is the macronutrient levels. Low-carb diets are considered any diet with a carb intake under about 100-150 grams of carbs per day. It's likely that you'll have to lower your carb intake much more to enter a state of ketosis.

The Atkins Diet is different from keto because of its different phases, which range from severely restricting carbs to adding a liberal amount of carbs (about 80-100 grams daily) back into the diet.

The keto diet works best when you stick to consistently low carb intake under about 50 grams per day for most people.

Difference In Protein Intake

Most low-carb diets are also high-protein diets. However, the keto diet ranges in protein intake, from moderate (around 20% of your total calories) to high-protein intake.

High-protein intake was once thought to spike blood sugar on a ketogenic diet, but there's evidence that you don't need to worry about gluconeogenesis as much as once thought. Still, diets like Atkins depend heavily on protein, without healthy, low-carb veggies for a majority of the diet.

If you're unsure of your optimal protein intake, check out the Keto Calculator to get your unique macronutrient guidelines.

Difference In Goals

The goals between these diets vary as well. The goal of keto is to enter ketosis, weaning your body off burning glucose for fuel for the long-term.

You may never enter ketosis with a low-carb diet. And although you may enter ketosis for a brief period on the Atkins Diet, you'll pop right back out in Phases 3 and 4 as you reintroduce higher levels of carbohydrate-rich foods.

Ketogenic Diet Macronutrients

Macronutrients seem to be the cornerstone of any keto diet, but contrary to popular opinion, there is no ONE macronutrient ratio that works for everyone.

Instead, you're going to have a completely different set of macros than your friend or your mother based on:

Your physical and mental goals Your

health history

Your activity level

The best way to figure these numbers out quickly is to refer to this macronutrient calculator.

Outside of your personal macros, there are general macro guidelines for a ketogenic diet:

70-80% of calories from fats

20-25% of calories from protein

5-10% of calories from carbohydrates

Below, these percentages are broken down into grams. Remember, these should be used as a guideline only. Your macronutrient goals will vary depending on your particular lifestyle.

Fat Intake

Fat is known as the cornerstone of the keto diet because fat does not raise your blood glucose like protein and carbs.

It was once thought that, in order to get into ketosis, you needed to eat massive amounts of fat on a daily basis. However, that's just not true.

The real secret to getting into ketosis is to cut carbs. You can modulate your fat intake from there. However, the accepted rule of thumb for most keto dieters is to stick to anywhere from 70-80% of your calories from healthy fats.

That means, if you're consuming 2,000 calories per day, you would need 144 to 177 grams of fat.

Protein Intake

Protein has gotten a bad rap in the keto community. Some experts claimed that eating too much protein on a very low-carb diet could trigger a metabolic effect called gluconeogenesis.

Protein is extremely important on the keto diet especially if you're active or an athlete.

Ideally, you should consume at least 0.8 grams of protein per pound of lean body mass to prevent muscle loss. For those of you with an extremely active lifestyle, 1 gram of protein per pound of lean body mass is ideal.

To calculate your lean body mass, you have to:

Calculate your body fat percentage. Click here to read how.

Subtract your body fat % from 100%. This will be your lean body mass %.

Multiply your lean body mass % by your total weight.

Or, you can check out the Keto Calculator to figure out your ideal protein intake.

So while most keto sites recommend 10-15% of total calories from protein, know that you can eat a lot more without raising your blood glucose or kicking you out of ketosis.

Carbohydrate Intake

Most people who want to get into ketosis should get about 5-10% of total calories from carbohydrates.

This usually looks like anywhere from 100-200 calories from carbs or about 25-50 grams of carbohydrates per day.

Most people consume roughly 30 grams of carbohydrates on the keto diet. Depending upon your activity level and health needs, you might be able to consume 80 grams of carbs and remain in ketosis.

Different Types of Ketogenic Diets

There are five main approaches to the ketogenic diet. When deciding which method works best for you, take into account your goals, fitness level, and what's realistic for your lifestyle.

The Standard Ketogenic Diet (Skd)

This is the most common and recommended version of the diet. Here, you stay within 20-50 grams of net carbs per day, focusing on moderate protein intake and high fat intake.

Targeted Ketogenic Diet (Tkd)

If you are an active individual, this approach might work best for you. Targeted keto involves eating roughly 25-50 grams of net carbs or less 30 minutes to an hour before exercise.

Cyclical Ketogenic Diet (CKD)

If keto seems intimidating to you, this is an excellent method to start with. You cycle between periods of eating a low-carb diet for several days, followed by a period of eating higher amounts of carbs (typically lasting several days).

High-Protein Ketogenic Diet (Hpkd)

This approach is very similar to the standard (SKD) approach. The primary difference is your protein intake. While a standard keto diet will include moderate protein, here you up your protein intake considerably.

Plant-Based Keto

Plant-based keto could range from eating more low-carb vegetables to going keto as a full-on vegan or vegetarian. You can follow the ketogenic diet as a vegetarian or as a vegan, but it will take a lot of work and effort to do this safely.

What Can You Eat on a Keto Diet?

Now that you understand the basics behind the keto diet, it's time to hit the grocery store.

On the keto diet, you'll enjoy nutrient-dense foods including meat, vegetables, nuts and seeds, and plenty of healthy fats.

You'll also avoid grains, legumes, processed foods, and most fruits. Consume these keto-friendly foods while staying within your macro guidelines:

Meat, Eggs, And Nuts

All meat and seafood are included on the keto diet, as long as they're, not breaded or fried.

Always choose the highest quality meat, you can afford, selecting grass-fed and organic beef whenever possible, wild-caught fish, and pasture-raised poultry, pork, and eggs.

Nuts and seeds are also fine and best eaten raw (not roasted or coated in sugar).

Enjoy:

Beef, preferably fattier cuts like steak, veal, roast, ground beef and stews

Poultry, including chicken breasts, quail, duck, turkey and wild game try to focus on the darker, fattier meats

Pork, including pork loin, tenderloin, chops, ham, and sugar-free bacon

Fish, including mackerel, tuna, salmon, trout, halibut, cod, catfish, and mahi-mahi

Shellfish, including oysters, clams, crab, mussels, and lobster

Organ meats, including heart, liver, tongue, kidney, and offal

Eggs, including deviled, fried, scrambled and boiled use the whole egg Lamb

Goat

Vegetarian sources, like macadamia nuts, almonds, and nut butter

Low-Carb Vegetables

On a keto meal plan, feel free to fill your plate with low-carb vegetables.

Vegetables are a great way to get a healthy dose of micronutrients, thus preventing vitamin deficiencies on keto.

Enjoy low-carb vegetables like leafy greens, and cruciferous veggies, aiming to eat veggies that contain fewer than 5 grams of net carbs per serving.

Enjoy these low carb vegetables:

Leafy greens, such as kale, spinach, swiss chard and arugula Cruciferous

vegetables, including cabbage, cauliflower, and zucchini Lettuces, including

iceberg, romaine, and butterhead

Fermented vegetables like sauerkraut and kimchi

Other vegetables such as mushrooms, asparagus, and celery

Keto-Friendly Dairy

If you can tolerate dairy, it is allowed on the keto diet. Choose the highest quality you can reasonably afford, selecting grass-fed, whole-fat, and organic dairy whenever possible.

Keto-friendly dairy options include: Butter

and ghee

Heavy cream and heavy whipping cream Fermented

dairy products like yogurts and kefir Sour cream

Hard and soft cheeses

Low-Sugar Fruits

Approach fruit with caution on keto, as it contains high amounts of sugar and carbohydrates. If you are craving something light and sweet, grab a handful of berries, such as blueberries or raspberries, as a treat.

Enjoy these low sugar fruits:

Avocadoes (the one fruit you can enjoy in abundance)

Organic berries, such as raspberries, blueberries, strawberries, and cranberries

Healthy Fats And Oils

You can enjoy both animal fats (saturated fats) and plant-based fats on a healthy keto diet.

Healthy fat sources include grass-fed butter, tallow, and ghee or coconut oil, olive oil, sustainable palm oil and MCT oil from plants.

Enjoy these fats and oils on keto: Butter

and ghee

Lard Mayonnaise

Coconut oil, coconut butter

Flaxseed oil

Olive oil Sesame seed

oil

MCT oil and MCT powder

Walnut oil

Olive oil, avocado oil

Herbs And Spices

Use seasonings freely on keto just make sure they don't have any added sugar. To add

flavor to dishes, consider purchasing fresh herbs at the store.

Pro tip: If you store fresh herbs in a mason jar filled with water in the fridge, they will last up to two weeks.

Foods to Avoid on a Keto Diet

It's best to avoid the following foods on a keto diet due to their high carb content.

When starting keto, do a purge of your fridge and cupboards. Donate any unopened items and throw the rest away.

Grains

Grains are loaded with carbs, so it's best to avoid all grains on keto. Whole grains, wheat, pasta, rice, oats, barley, rye, corn, and quinoa are all out. Instead, try one of these substitutes.

Beans And Legumes

While many vegans and vegetarians rely beans for their protein content, they are actually incredibly high-carb. Avoid eating kidney beans, chickpeas, black beans, and lentils.

Higher-Sugar Fruits

While many fruits are packed with antioxidants and other micronutrients, they're also high in fructose, which will kick you out of ketosis.

Avoid apples, mangos, pineapple and other fruits (with the exception of small amounts of berries).

Starchy Veggies

Avoid starchy vegetables like potatoes, sweet potatoes, some squash, parsnips, and carrots.

Like fruit, there are health benefits to these foods. However, you can find those vitamins and minerals from low-carb sources ones that won't kick you out of ketosis.

Sugar

This includes, but is not limited to desserts, artificial sweeteners, smoothies, soda, and fruit juice.

Even condiments like ketchup and BBQ sauce are usually filled with sugar, so put down the ketchup bottle. If you are craving a dessert, try one of these keto-friendly recipes instead.

Alcohol

Some alcoholic beverages are low-glycemic and appropriate for a ketogenic diet. However, keep in mind that when you drink alcohol, your liver will preferentially process the ethynol and stop producing ketones.

If you're on a ketogenic diet to lose weight, keep your alcohol consumption to a minimum. If you're craving a cocktail, stick to low-sugar mixers and avoid most beer and wine.

Seed Oils

Seed oils are heavily processed and can become oxidized (aka, rancid) when you heat them. Avoid corn oil, canola oil, peanut oil, and grapeseed oil. They also contain large amounts of omega–6 fatty acids, which are inflammatory in large amounts.

Health Benefits of a Keto Diet

A ketogenic diet has been associated with incredible health benefits that stretch way beyond weight loss. Here are just a few ways keto may help you feel better, stronger, and more clear-headed:

Keto For Weight Loss

Probably what the keto diet is most famous for: sustainable fat loss. Keto can significantly decrease body weight, body fat, and body mass while maintaining muscle mass. Keto can also increase fat metabolism during exercise, making it an excellent part of your active lifestyle.

Keto For Endurance Levels

The ketogenic diet may help improve endurance levels for athletes. However, it may take time for athletes to adjust to burning fat instead of glucose for energy.

Keto For Gut Health

Several studies have shown a link between low sugar intake and improvement in symptoms of irritable bowel syndrome (IBS). In fact, one study showed that eating a ketogenic diet can improve abdominal pain and overall quality of life in those with IBS.

Keto For Diabetes

The ketogenic diet helps to balance blood sugar and insulin levels, which helps immensely with metabolic diseases like type 2 diabetes.

Keto For Heart Health

The keto diet can help reduce risk factors for heart disease, including improvement in HDL cholesterol, triglycerides, and LDL cholesterol (related to plaque in the arteries).

Keto For Brain Health

The keto diet may support those with Parkinson's, Alzheimer's disease, and other degenerative brain diseases This is likely because ketone bodies having possible neuroprotective and anti-inflammatory benefits.

Keto For Skin Health

Because ketones and lower blood sugar contribute to overall hormone balance and lower inflammatory markers, the keto diet may be good for skin health. One study suggests that decreased skin inflammation can decrease acne and other skin lesions.

Keto For Epilepsy

The ketogenic diet was created in the early 20th century to help prevent seizures in epileptic patients, especially children. To this day, ketosis is a go-to therapeutic diet for those who suffer from epilepsy.

Keto For Cancer Support

There's a growing body of research that suggests a strict keto diet can help slow tumor growth. Although no one diet can cure or prevent cancer, a low-carb, zero-sugar diet is a great place to start.

Keto For Pms

An estimated 90% of women experience one or more of symptoms associated with PMS. A keto diet can help balance blood sugar, combat chronic inflammation, boost your nutrient stores, and crush cravings all of which may help alleviate your PMS symptoms.

How to Know When You're in Ketosis

You can follow the above macronutrient guidelines, eat the prescribed keto diet foods and avoid grains, starches, and legumes and still struggle to enter ketosis.

Why? Because ketosis is a metabolic state, and you may need to tweak your meal plan, exercise regimen, and other lifestyle choices in order to enter it.

There are plenty of signs and symptoms to suggest you're in ketosis, including: Weight

loss

Fewer cravings Better

mental clarity More stable

energy

But there's only one reliable way to know whether or not you're in ketosis: Test your ketone levels.

There are three ways to do this: In your

urine with a urine strip

In your blood with a glucose meter On your

breath with a breath meter

The Ketogenic Diet Heirarchy of Needs Testing

Each method has its advantages and disadvantages, with a blood test being the most accurate (but most expensive). Although it's the most affordable, urine testing is typically the least accurate method.

Supplements to Support a Keto Diet

Supplements are a popular way to maximize the benefits of a ketogenic diet. You can't get all of your nutrients from supplements and expect to feel good, but they can help.

Add in these supplements alongside a healthy, whole-food based keto diet for the best results.

Exogenous Ketones

"Exogenous ketones" are supplemental ketones usually beta-hydroxybutyrate or acetoacetate that help kick you into ketosis and give you the energy you need to thrive. You can take exogenous ketones in between meals or for a quick burst of energy before a workout.

MCT Oil And Powder

MCTs (or medium-chain triglycerides) are a type of fatty acid that your body can convert to energy quickly and efficiently. Benefits includes weight loss and energy, among other things. MCTs come from coconuts and are sold mostly in liquid form. Perfect Keto sells them as a delicious and easy-to-use powder.

Collagen Protein

Collagen is the most abundant protein in your body, accounting for about 25-35%. It's the glue that holds your body together as it supports the growth of joints, organs, hair, and connective tissues. Amino acids from collagen supplements may also help with energy production, DNA repair, detox, and healthy digestion.

Micronutrient Supplements

It's tough to get all the micronutrients you need from diet alone regardless of what nutrition regimen you're on. Keto Micro Greens is the solution to getting all your micronutrients in one convenient scoop.

Ketogenic Pre-Workout Supplements

Keto pre-workout supplements like Perfect Keto Perform Pre-Workout can boost physical and cognitive performance without the caffeine crash. It contains exogenous ketones and MCT oil powder for energy, creatine for protein metabolism, branched- chain amino acids for muscle growth and repair, and more.

Whey Protein

One of the best-studied supplements for weight loss support, muscle gain and maintenance, and recovery. Make sure to choose grass-fed whey only and avoid powders with sugar or any other additives that could spike blood sugar.

Electrolytes

Electrolyte balance is one of the most critical yet most overlooked components of a successful ketogenic diet experience. Especially when you're just starting out. A keto diet can make you excrete more electrolytes than usual so you have to replenish them yourself. Add more sodium, potassium, and calcium to your diet or grab a supplement that can help.

Krill Oil

Get even more of the benefits of an anti-inflammatory keto diet with some high-quality omega-3 fatty acids. Krill oil is just as potent as fish oil, without the fishy aftertaste. Krill also contains phospholipids and a potent antioxidant called astaxanthin that fish oil doesn't.

Blood Sugar Support

Think about adding vitamins, minerals, and herbs to support normal digestion, metabolism, hormone function, and energy production. Take these with higher carb meals to support healthy carbohydrate metabolism or just to promote healthy nutrient absorption.

Is the Ketogenic Diet Safe?

Ketosis is a perfectly safe and natural metabolic state, but it is often confused with a highly dangerous metabolic state called ketoacidosis.

Having ketone levels in the 0.5-5.0mmol/L range is not dangerous, but other risks include a range of issues, from harmless keto flu symptoms to diabetic ketoacidosis, which is not a problem unless you're diabetic.

Ketoacidosis

Diabetic ketoacidosis (DKA) is a dangerous metabolic state that is most commonly seen in people with type 1 diabetes and sometimes type 2 diabetics if they aren't properly managing their insulin and diet.

Keto Flu Symptoms

Many people deal with common side effects similar to flu-like symptoms as they become fat adapted after decades of running on carbs. These temporary symptoms are byproducts of dehydration and low carbohydrate levels while your body adjusts:

Headaches

Lethargy Nausea

Brain fog

Stomach pain Low

motivation

The keto flu can often be shortened or avoided completely by taking one of our ketone supplements, which help switch the body into ketosis instantly. They make the transition period much shorter and easier.

Different Types of Ketogenic Diets

Over the past several years, people have found different ways to approach the ketogenic diet.

Depending on your goals and fitness level, you may find one type of keto diet fits your lifestyle better than others. No matter which one you choose, the goal should be to shift your body from using carbs to using fat as your primary source of fuel.

Here's a breakdown of the different type of keto diets:

Standard Ketogenic Diet (Skd)

This is the most straightforward approach to the ketogenic diet. On the SKD, you're keeping your total carbs extremely low while focusing most of your macronutrient intake on fat and protein. The goal of SKD is to get into and maintain a state of ketosis, burning fat as your primary source of fuel.

Cyclical Ketogenic Diet (CKD)

The cyclical ketogenic diet is a good choice if your goal is to increase muscle strength and improve exercise performance. When following the CKD you're cycling days of ketosis with days of higher carb intake. A typical CKD will be five to six days eating a keto diet (very low-carb), with one or two days of higher carb intake.

The purpose is to reap the benefits of keto during the days on, and on the re-feeding carb days to restore your glycogen stores for huge amounts of activity.

As mentioned earlier, glucose from carbs is a very readily available source of fuel. For athletes and bodybuilders, this can be a great way to get the best of both worlds.

Targeted Ketogenic Diet(Tkd)

The TKD is similar to the standard ketogenic diet, with the exception that you can eat carbohydrates around (before or after) heavy workouts. This approach is for you if you're performing high-intensity workouts for extended periods of time.

If you exercise regularly and are burning fuel at a significant rate, this may be a good strategy for you. Especially if you find yourself "bonking" during workouts when you're in ketosis.

Some athletes notice a decrease in stamina after they've switched to keto.

This approach allows them to benefit from the rapid fuel source of glucose, while also burning it up quickly enough to get back into a ketogenic state. This strategy is best for people who are working out for an hour or more at a moderate to high intensity.

High-Protein Ketogenic Diet

The high-protein keto diet is becoming popular as more people are discovering that they can eat higher protein while still maintaining a ketogenic state.

A high-protein ketogenic diet should be around 30-35% protein, with 60% fat, keeping carbs just as low as you would on a standard ketogenic diet.

This is a good option for people who are active and want to maintain muscle mass. It's also an approach to play with if you're having a hard time sticking to a very high-fat, low- to moderate-protein diet.

Regardless of your macronutrient ratio, the goal is to maintain a ketogenic state for as much of the time as possible, so you can reap all the benefits of being in a ketogenic state.

Benefits of a Keto Diet

Many anecdotal accounts of the keto diet claim rapid weight loss, better brain function, and fewer food cravings. But there are plenty of scientifically-backed benefits of the keto diet as well. Here are just a few:

Blood Sugar Control

Studies have found that people with type 2 diabetes do exceptionally well on a ketogenic diet. Studies show that the extreme reduction in carbs showed an increase in blood glucose control as well as a reduced need for insulin controlling medication.

Fat Loss

Despite higher caloric intake, the ketogenic diet is superior to a low-fat diet for fat loss. Fat loss around the midsection (metabolically active fat) seems to be a specific target in ketogenic fat loss.

Mental Clarity

Many people report feeling enhanced mental sharpness and clarity when following a ketogenic diet. Part of this response may come from higher energy utilization along with the anti-inflammatory effect of the ketogenic diet.

Blood Lipid Profile

Following a ketogenic diet can improve your blood lipid profile. Specifically, it can increase HDL (good cholesterol) and also increase the size of your LDL particles. Larger, fluffier LDL particles are safer because they are less likely to contribute to plaques.

Lower Inflammation

One of the three ketone bodies, beta-hydroxybutyrate (BHB), has been shown to decrease inflammation in your body by blocking an inflammatory signaling pathway.

Heart Disease

Due to its positive effect on both blood lipids and inflammation, the ketogenic diet may benefit those with or at risk for heart disease.

Neurological Disease

The ketogenic diet has been used for over 80 years to treat epilepsy, a disorder in which the nerve cell activity in your brain is disturbed, leading to seizures.

14 DAY KETO DIET MENU FOR BEGINNERS

WEEK 1:
MONDAY
Breakfast: Cheesy Keto Bagels
Lunch: Zesty Chili Lime Keto Tuna Salad
Dinner: Nutritious Baked Pork Chops

TUESDAY
Breakfast: Avocado Egg Bowls
Lunch: Low-Carb Romanesco with Cabbage Noodles
Dinner: One-Pan Cheesy Broccoli Chicken Casserole
WEDNESDAY
Breakfast: Breakfast Casserole with Bacon, Egg, and Cheese Lunch:
Grass-Fed Keto Beef Bulgogi
Dinner: Lemon Balsamic Chicken

THURSDAY
Breakfast: Cinnamon Dolce Latte Breakfast Smoothie Lunch: Spicy
Ginger Salmon Buddha Bowl
Dinner: Loaded Cauliflower Bake

FRIDAY
Breakfast: Almond Flour Low-Carb Crepes Lunch:
Crispy Parmesan Crusted Chicken
Dinner: Crispy Skin Salmon With Pesto Cauliflower Rice

SATURDAY
Breakfast: Savory Breakfast Keto Sausage Balls Lunch:
Portobello Bun Cheeseburgers
Dinner: Keto Chicken Cordon Blue

SUNDAY
Breakfast: Chocolate Protein Pancakes Lunch:
Keto Low-Carb Chili
Dinner: Stuffed Keto Pork Loin

WEEK 2: MONDAY
Breakfast: Keto N'oatmeal
Lunch: Spicy Low-Carb Salmon Patties
Dinner: Low-Carb Keto Pot Roast

TUESDAY
Breakfast: Turkey Sausage Frittata
Lunch: Rich and Creamy Keto Broccoli Cheese Soup Dinner: Spicy
Grass-Fed Keto Fajitas

WEDNESDAY
Breakfast: Smoked Salmon Keto Avocado Toast Lunch:
Easy Keto Chicken Salad
Dinner: Keto Grass-Fed Beef Stew

THURSDAY
Breakfast: Pumpkin Cream Cheese Muffins Lunch:
Zesty Keto Taco Salad
Dinner: Tender Keto Pork Chops

FRIDAY
Breakfast: Micronutrient Greens Matcha Smoothie Lunch:
Curry Chicken Lettuce Wraps
Dinner: Fathead Pizza: Low-Carb Keto Pizza

SATURDAY
Breakfast: Keto Egg Muffins
Lunch: Low-Carb Cauliflower Mac and Cheese Dinner:
Delicious Low-Carb Keto Meatloaf

SUNDAY
Breakfast: Fluffy Salted Caramel Pumpkin Spice Pancakes Lunch:
Savory Shrimp Keto Stir-Fry
Dinner: Low-Carb Keto Lasagna

Dessert Options:
Indulgent Keto Peanut Butter Cups
Creamy Chocolate No Churn Keto Ice Cream Thick
and Rich Keto Whipped Cream Matcha Chia Seed
Pudding
Chocolate Sea Salt Peanut Butter Bites
Rich and Creamy Pumpkin Spice Keto Mocha

PROS AND CONS OF KETOGENIC DIETING

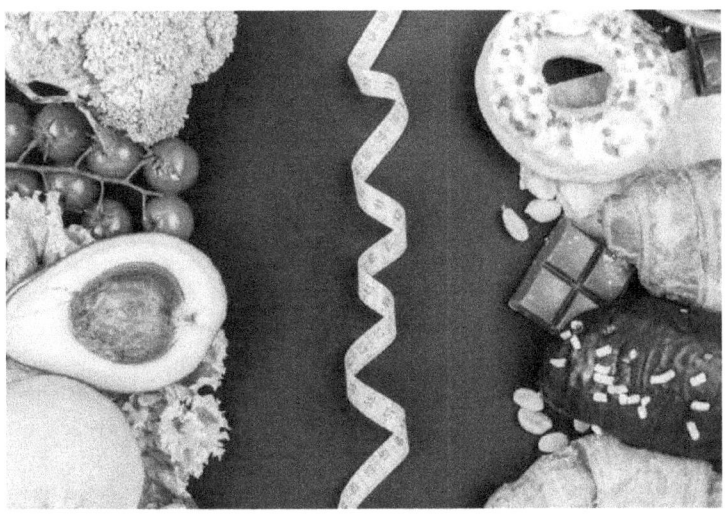

The Atkins diet itself is only the most popular of an approach usually called low-carb diets because of the primary interest in restricting consumption of Carbohydrates. Since the entire spectrum of our food is drawn from proteins, fats, carbohydrates or water, severe restriction of one group is seen by many as an arbitrary and possibly even dangerous step.

Most of the controversy surrounding low-carb approaches is not that they lie about weight-loss (studies continue to show marked weight-loss in many who use the diets) but the disturbing possibility that cutting the carbs out of your diet just isn't healthy. After all, what good is a diet that slims you down only to clog up your arteries and kill you? We've heard many arguments both for and against the use of low-carbohydrate diets, this article asks a radical question: Can going Low-Carb actually be healthy?

Why Should I Limit Sugar & Grains?

The first and most obvious carbohydrate group and one we rarely have much argument about reducing is sugar. Sugar is a catch all term for a number of simple carbohydrates including fructose (fruit sugar), Galactose (milk sugar), sucrose (table sugar) and glucose (simple sugars such as blood sugar). Sugar consumption has been on the increase for decades and, despite the numerous campaigns against saturated fats, is certainly the biggest contributing factor to the increasing obesity epidemic.

Eating sugar causes a number of physiological effects in the body. The most striking of these is the sudden and marked increase in blood insulin. Insulin is the hormone in our body responsible for 'taxiing' the food broken down in out stomach to the various parts of our body that require these substances, although it has numerous uses. First, and most importantly, sugar, as glucose levels in out blood is extremely toxic. Left in our bloodstream without control elevated sugar levels would kill us quickly, so the powerful release of insulin helps keep our blood cleared of excess glucose. Unfortunately insulin is a double-edged sword. Excess sugar in our body cannot be disposed of in an unlimited number of ways. With our increasing sedentary lifestyles refusing to burn off much of this sudden and quick release of carbohydrate as we consume, sugar is rapidly converted to the same saturated fats we are constantly warned about. (As you can see, limiting saturated fat in the diet does not prevent us from accumulating fat in our bodies).

Sugar has other unpleasant side effects. The constantly elevated insulin levels can eventually lead to decreased insulin sensitivity (Syndrome X) and another case of Type II diabetes. Sugar also has an effect on cortisol and our adrenal glands. It causes an excess of these hormones leading to symptoms of stress and fatigue. Sugar also competes with the glucose carriers in our blood, which work with vitamins like Vitamin C, causing disruption to our preciously balanced immune system and causing premature ageing of the skin.

Sugar can be thought of as nitro-fuel for the body. It releases a very quick but harsh burst of artificial energy. Inactive individuals requiring peak performance from athletic pursuits, simple carbohydrates can be a useful tool, especially in the area of pre and post workout drinks. Much like a drag-racer using nitro fuel, this substance can be used to replace muscle glycogen and spare muscle wastage due to overtraining effects. Unfortunately few of us use sugar in this careful and controlled manner and are attempting to drive the finely balanced engines of our bodies on a fuel which causes too much stress and strain on a system that was never designed to handle the excess we provide.

So since low-carb diets almost completely eliminate sugar from our diets, we have already found one significant health benefit.

Grain Controversy

Most of our Western Governments offer health guidelines which ask us to base our food intake almost universally around grain-type carbohydrates, what were once grouped as starches. We know these most commonly as rice, pasta, potatoes and breads. These types of food appear to have been staples of our western diets since time immemorial (they're not, but that's another story). We are often told that eating these foods will leave us full, satisfied and full of a slow releasing stream of energy that is healthy and safe. Unfortunately, at least for human beings, this doesn't always appear to be the case.

Not all grains are created equal for a start and this can be where grain advocates purposely or accidentally mislead. For instance most rice, particularly white rice, will convert to sugar almost immediately in our system and we've already seen some of the devastating effects of excess sugar consumption. Grains, no matter what source they come from will cause elevated insulin levels. For the very healthy amongst us, who have extremely sensitive insulin (either through good genetics, regular exercise or a combination of both) may be able to carefully use small quantities of grains to fuel their bodies through the periods of high activity. However for the vast majority of people, the excess of grains will result in almost all the same problems as sugar consumption. Many low-carb exponents are suspicious of medical advice to eat grains, many citing

Government subsidies of mass agriculture. Eating grains is a very cheap and simple way of providing food, but cheap and simple is rarely the same as healthy and good.

Vegetables!

Low carb diets have often been seen as lacking in vegetables as people carefully trim away all excess carbohydrates, effectively throwing the baby out with the dirty bathwater. On the subject of vegetables, you won't find much dissension amongst medical experts of any standpoint. These wonderful foodstuffs not only contain a plethora of vitamins and minerals, but also are often chock-full of fiber, water and a host of exotic cancer-fighting substances unique to vegetables.

The important thing about vegetables are is that they are nutrient dense and calorie sparse. In plain English, they contain a lot of good stuff in a very small package. You can eat virtually enough vegetables to fill you up and still have eaten only a tiny percentage of the calories a normal diet would confer.

One of the arguments for regular grain consumption is the necessary vitamins and minerals they contain, not to mention the essential fibre for our digestive tract. But guess what? Vegetables makes grains seem pretty redundant. A small handful of organic vegetables will contain more vitamins and minerals than virtually a day's worth of grains, all in an easier to digest package, with extra water and no danger of insulin overload.

Even on a low-carb diet you can stuff yourself silly with vegetables without fear. The primary advantage of a low-carb diet is insulin control and vegetables won't interfere with that. Remember organic vegetables have a much higher vitamin and mineral content, also the darker green or red a vegetable the higher the amount of beneficial Chlorophyll inside the plant. Try to eat your veggies raw and fresh and often. A regular supply of varied veggies is like nature's most perfect multivitamin pill.

Eat Veggies But

What About All The Other Foods You Need?

So low-carb dieters are shedding the pounds by avoiding the insulin spiking grains and sugars. In the process they're moving over to eating other stuff though right? You stop eating bread and pasta and you've got to eat something! We see Atkins dieters especially loading up proteins and fats, burgers, sausages, bacon, full double cream, fried eggs and a host of other tasty but controversial foods. So, fine, we can accept that somehow these people still seem to shed weight much faster and more consistently than their carbohydrate munching friends but surely, surely, that can't be HEALTHY?

Too good to be true? Some Doctors definitely believe so. We've been warned about saturated fat and our rising cholesterol problem for a number of years. Suddenly a diet comes along that seems to throw all that conventional wisdom out of the window.

As it happens, the American Medical Association was forced to declare the Atkins diet 'heart-healthy' after a number of university studies came up with the surprising findings that Atkins dieters were actually lowering their blood fat deposits and sparing the hearts much more than those on a regular higher carb diet.

First we know the basis of that diet is our good friend, the organic vegetable. But moving on, it seems our bodies were designed for a much greater range of essential nutrients than those found in vegetable alone. First up Fats. Yes, it may have finally begun to infiltrate the mainstream press but its old news to many of us. Fat is essential! We need to eat fat. There's no getting around it, our bodies don't merely tolerate the stuff, they absolutely need it to function. When you remember that our brains are over sixty percent fat, our organs require it and our very nerves are built from it, you begin to see how important it is. However much like our friend the Carbohydrate, all fats are not created equal either. Our bodies need a small group of fats that we call 'Essential Fatty Acids'. Our body cannot produce these from any other substances and needs a regular supply or it begins to see shortcomings in its internal workings. We can get by for a while on diminished supplies but our health begins to suffer greatly in the long run.

These healthy fats come in the form of the well-publicised fish and cod-liver oils, flax and various other nut oils and foods like avocado. (Although not essential organic coconut oil has a host of special benefits) Simply be ensuring that a large percentage of our daily fat intake comes from clean, healthy oils will go a long way to improving our health, from defending our brain against degenerative diseases to protecting our skin from the harmful rays of the sun. To be a healthy low carber you need to investigate healthy fats a little more and remember that high quality, preferably organic oils are a better choice than others. There are a host of books on this subject and a host of great products out there. Unfortunately due to the mass pollution of the seas, fish may no longer be the healthiest option, although carefully filtrated fish-oils (by Companies who are clued up on the science of keeping these oils in a health-giving state) are widely available and a must-buy for everyone.

Protein covers the widest range of foods left to us. Protein, which makes up our body's muscles, can be found from the flesh of other animals as well as from milks, beans and lentils. Much like fat, our body requires protein. How much is open to debate. Active individuals, particularly those who require larger muscles, will have a much higher protein need than a sedentary individual but sufficed to say, excess protein intake (although feared by many mainstream nutritionists) has none of the dangers that excess grain or sugar consumption does.

That said, we could always make healthier choices. Although the Atkins diet may allow us to eat burgers and bacon all day long, this may not be the ideal choice. When considering meat products we have to remember what state the animal it came from was in when it was slaughtered. Most animals in large factory farming business are over-fed, over medicated cripples and surely this meat can't be entirely healthy. Foods like bacon also contain a large number of hazardous preservative chemicals that sap at our besieged immune systems. Once again, not all proteins are created equal. Choosing organic fresh meats from leaner animals is a wise choice when considering health.

Chicken and Turkey, from good organic sources is a lean and easy to use protein source. Animals such as bison (buffalo) and Ostrich may sound like exotic food sources to many, but their meat is almost entirely free from chemicals and their natural diets of grass and other non-artificial feeds leaves them with a low-fat content of good, healthy fats. High quality protein is essential to your health and survival. Eating lower-quality meats may allow you to stay trim (since protein consumption appears to regulate our appetite much better than grains ever could) but investing in higher quality meats will mean you can claim the health benefits as well.

The Healthy Low Carb Approach

As many low-carb dieters have pointed out, most humans were never designed to live on a high carbohydrate content in their diets. As hunter-gatherers we consisted mostly on animals that roamed wild and on fresh vegetables and berries we could find in our local habitat. Although our societies may have advanced enough to let us devise sustained agriculture, our genes are still locked in a hundred thousand-year-old struggle for survival. Our bodies recognise the nutrients available from clean meats, healthy fats and fresh vegetables. They have substantial trouble coping with the sudden influx of excess energy and too quickly absorbed carbohydrates in the form of grains and sugars.

Restricting the intake of grains and sugars makes a fairly quick and positive change towards a healthier life. However, it may be that, in our urge to shed the pounds with as little pain as possible, the lower carb diets we choose are tilted towards the proteins and fats we don't really need and attention to vegetables is ignored. With a few minor modifications we can find a lower-carbohydrate approach that not only helps us maintain a normalised body-weight and fat mass but also helps us be an all round healthier individual. There are a hundred other points towards improving health but all these changes make an admirable start.

KETOSIS SIDE EFFECTS

There are many awesome benefits with come with adopting a low-carb ketogenic diet, such as weight loss, decreased cravings, and even possibly reduce diseases risks. That being said, it's also good to talk about possible ketosis side effects so you know fully what to expect as you start this new health journey.

Common Ketosis Side Effects and Treatments

Not everyone experiences side effects when starting a ketogenic diet, and thankfully, those who do don't usually experience them for very long. It varies with the individual, but just to make sure all your bases are covered, we're going to breaking down each possible side effect and go over ways to manage and alleviate them if needed.

- – FREQUENT URINATION

As your body burns through the stored glucose in your liver and muscles within the first day or two of starting a ketogenic diet, you'll be releasing a lot of water in the process. Plus, your kidneys will start excreting excess sodium as the levels of your circulating insulin drop.

Basically, you might notice yourself needing to pee more often throughout the day. But no worries; this side effect of ketosis takes care of itself once your body adjusts and is no longer burning through the extra glycogen.

- – DIZZINESS AND DROWSINESS

As the body is getting rid of this excess water, it will also be eliminating minerals like potassium, magnesium, and sodium too. This can make you feel dizzy, lightheaded, and fatigued.

Thankfully, this is also very avoidable; all it takes is a little preparation beforehand. Focus on eating foods that are rich in potassium, such as:

Leafy greens (aim for at least two cups each day!)

Broccoli

Dairy

Meat, poultry, and fish

Avocados

Add salt to your foods or use salty broth when cooking too. You can also dissolve about a teaspoon of regular salt in a glass of water and increase your hydration at the same time.

Adding salt to food might be new to you, since most people are used to being told to limit salt intake. However, when you're eating a ketogenic diet of less than 60 carbohydrates each day, you'll need to make up for this loss of salt. That being said, those with high blood pressure who take medication should check with their doctors before making a change.

- – LOW BLOOD SUGAR

Also known as hypoglycemia, low blood sugar is another common ketosis side effect when beginning a ketogenic diet, especially for people who were used to eating higher amounts of carbs each day. When your body is used to intaking more carbs, it becomes accustomed to putting a certain amount of insulin out to handle the sugar.

So, when the amount of sugar intake is drastically reduced on a keto diet, it's possible to experience short-term episodes of low blood sugar. That can make you feel temporarily tired, hungry, or shaky until your body adjusts.

– – CRAVINGS FOR SUGAR

A great long-term benefit of the ketogenic diet is reduced cravings for sugar and other unhealthy foods. However, you might initially have stronger cravings for carbs during the transition period. This can last anywhere from one to two days to around three weeks. But stick it out! At the end, you'll be pleased with the reduced, and often eliminated, cravings.

– – CONSTIPATION

As your digestive system adapts, you might initially experience some constipation when new to the keto diet. This is often caused by dehydration as you release more fluids (remember how we talked about going to the bathroom more?).

Remedy constipation by making sure your intake of fiber is high, eating tons of non- starchy vegetables, getting enough salt, and drink tons of water each day to moisten the contents of the colon.

If that doesn't help completely, try cutting back on your nut and dairy consumption. You might also consider taking 400 mg of magnesium citrate.

– – DIARRHEA

On the flip side of the previously mentioned side effect, some people might experience minor issues with diarrhea in the first few days. This can simply be a result of your body adjusting to the macronutrient ratio change. In other cases, some people make the mistake of limiting their fat intake along with their carbs, which makes your intake of protein too high and can lead to diarrhea.

Don't skip on your fats! Be sure the carbs you're limiting are being replaced by full fat sources instead of proteins.

- - MUSCLE CRAMPS

Loss of minerals when first starting the keto diet can cause muscle cramps, especially leg cramps, in some people. Like with other side effects we've mentioned, drinking lots of water and eating salt can help by preventing cramps and reducing mineral loss.

- - FLU-LIKE SYMPTOMS

Within the first 2-4 days of beginning a keto diet, a common side effect is known as the "ketosis flu" or "induction flu" because it mimics the symptoms of an actual flu. This means you might experience:

Headaches

Tiredness or lack of motivation

Lethargy

Brain fog or confusion

Irritability

Although these symptoms typically go away completely within a few days, they are also completely avoidable if you stay very hydrated and increase your salt intake (seeing a pattern here?). And like always, be sure you're eating enough fat.

- - SLEEP ISSUES

Some people have reported having trouble sleeping after beginning a ketogenic diet. If this sounds like you, it could mean your serotonin and insulin levels are low.

Try having a snack right before you go to bed that contains protein as well as some carbs to increase insulin and give your brain a nice dose of tryptophan, which is the precursor for serotonin, from the protein.

Another possible reason for impaired sleep could be increased intake of food rich in histamines, which can cause more anxiety and sleeplessness in some people. You can remedy this by eating less cheeses, avocado, bacon, and eggs, which contain a lot of histamines, and replacing them with more vegetables in your diet.

- – SMELLY BREATH

Some people experience the smell of acetone on their breath when eating very low carb. Acetone is one of the ketone bodies created during ketosis, and it has a characteristically fruity smell similar to nail polish remover. This is a sign your body is in ketosis, burning lots of fats and converting them to ketones for energy. That's great news!

Plus, those who notice this smell on their breath or body (and not everyone does) report it usually going away within 1-2 weeks as the body adapts to ketosis. But if it doesn't completely go away in this amount of time, here are some tips for resolving it:

Keep good oral hygiene. Keep your breath fresh by brushing your teeth well at least twice day (hopefully you're doing this already!).

Increase water intake. Bad breath can be caused by less saliva from dry mouth as your body releases water in a low-carb state. Drinking plenty of water will help counteract this.

Use breath freshener. Although this won't eliminate the fruity smell completely, it will mask it as you wait for it to subside.

Slightly increase carbs. If you wait a few more weeks and still have trouble with the ketone smell, you might consider eating slightly more carbs to reduce the ketosis. Try increasing to between 50 and 70 grams per day. You might also try combining this with intermittent fasting, such as only eating within an 8-hour window, to maintain the benefits of ketosis without the side effect of fruity breath.

- – HEART PALPITATIONS

In the first few weeks of eating low carb, you might notice a slight increase in heart rate. This is probably more common in those who normally have low blood pressure.

It's often simply due to lack of salt and water, causing a reduction in the fluid circulating in the blood. This may then cause the heart to pump slightly faster or harder. So again, drink, drink, drink, and salt your foods!

This problem should go away within a week or two, but if you need to after that time, you can slightly increase your amount of carbs.

You might also want to consider a high-quality multivitamin containing zinc and selenium and a magnesium supplement to replace any nutrients lost during adaptation.

Caution For Those With Diabetes

People with diabetes should note that drastically reducing carbs can decrease the need for medicine taken to lower raised blood sugar, so taking the same amount of insulin as before could possible result in too-low blood sugar on a low-carb diet. Heart palpitations is a symptom of that.

Be sure to speak with your doctor about changes you might need to make, and test your sugar levels frequently when starting the diet.

Caution for Those with High Blood Pressure

Similar to diabetes medication, those with high blood pressure might notice that their dose becomes too strong after starting a low-carb diet, as it can improve blood pressure. Heart palpitations can also be a sign of this. Speak with your doctor about the changes and be sure to check your blood pressure at home too.

Reduced Physical Performance

You'll likely notice a large change in physical performance when first starting a low-carb way of eating, which is often caused by dehydration, lack of salt, and your body adjusting to burning fat for fuel.

It can take weeks and sometimes months for the body to adapt to the change from burning glucose for energy to using primarily fat. This part is mostly just a waiting game, but exercising while in transition might also help your body adapt faster.

Athletes are starting to experiment more with the long-term physical performance benefits of a low-carb diet, mostly those who do endurance sports and long-distance running, because there might be real advantages in performance once the body is keto- adapted. You can read more about the ketogenic diet for physical performance here.

SIDE EFFECTS OF USING A KETOGENIC DIET FOR WEIGHT LOSS

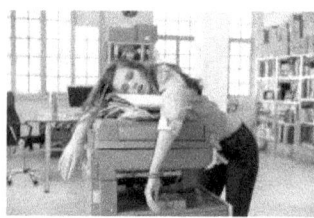

Keto Flu

This is one thing that anyone starting a ketogenic diet should brace up for. It is a condition in which you experience some of the different side effects that come along with using a ketogenic diet.

Keto flu is often characterized by light-headedness or brain fogginess, headaches, nausea, stomachaches, and muscle soreness. You may also experience heightened feelings of lethargy, irritability and trouble concentrating.

Interestingly, these are all common symptoms of the flu, hence the name. These symptoms are temporary and not everyone using a ketogenic is affected by them.

These symptoms are often caused by the sugar withdrawal occasioned by the significantly reduced carbohydrate intake. Also, an imbalance in your body electrolytes such as calcium, magnesium, potassium, and sodium can affect how your body reacts to the effect of a ketogenic diet.

Keto Breath

There are two possible reasons put forth why people on ketogenic diets experience this peculiar breath issue.

The body does not store ketones and thus they must be excreted from the body. Ketones can be excreted through the urine as acetoacetate.

They can also be excreted through the breath in form of acetone. So the more ketones you produce, the more acetone you pass out through your breath. Unfortunately, this can cause unpleasant-smelling breath when using a ketogenic diet.

On the other hand, increased protein ingestion can also cause keto breath. This is because the way the body digest fats and proteins is quite different. The digestion of proteins usually produces ammonia which the body excretes through the urine.

However, the increased consumption of proteins may result in the indigestible amounts remaining in your gut system and undergoes fermentation. This produces ammonia which is subsequently released through your breath.

Keto breath can last for about a week to just under a month. It is mostly depends on how well your body adapts to ketosis.

Micronutrient Deficiencies

This may result from the strict restrictions on carbohydrate intake. A lot of carbohydrate-rich foods are equally rich in vitamins and minerals.

The severe restriction on carbohydrate intake may therefore cause deficiencies in some essential nutrients. Therefore, we should not only be focused on the micronutrient counting in terms of fat, proteins, and carbohydrates but should also remember the vitamin and mineral micronutrient contents as well.

This is often why supplements are mostly recommended when using a ketogenic diet. Supplementation will help to augment any micronutrient imbalance that might occur when using a ketogenic diet.

AVOIDING Ketosis Side Effects

If you noticed the common theme in most of these side effects with the ketogenic diet, it involves the transition in and out of ketosis. This is one of the main reasons we have made Perfect Keto Base to eliminate any of the possible side effects as possible and ease the transition into ketosis.

The common ketosis side effects can be helped or eliminated by: drinking

more water

increasing your salt intake

and making sure you're eating enough fat

If you do still struggle with symptoms, though, a last resort would be to slightly increase the amount of carbs you're eating to alleviate symptoms. The downside to this is that it will make your low-carb diet effective less quickly, but sometimes that's necessary to continue it over the long-term.

HOW TO LOSE WEIGHT ON A KETOGENIC DIET

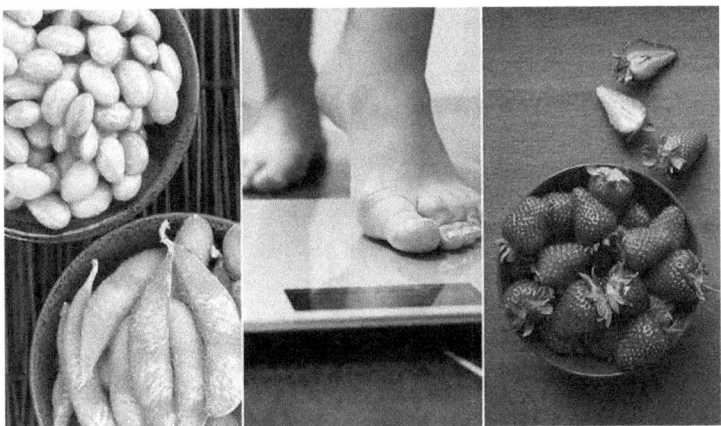

There are many ways to lose weight, and following the ketogenic diet is one of them. In fact, keto is one of the most effective ways to lose weight rapidly and keep the fat off for good.

This doesn't mean, that a high-fat, low-carb diet is ideal for everyone that is aiming for weight loss. Some people may fare better with other dietary choices that fit more snuggly into their current lifestyles.

Either way, it is possible for you to lose weight and keep it off. In this article, we will look at the research to find the most effective weight loss methods so that you can finally find something that works for you. But first, let's get a better grasp on the issue of obesity and its potential causes.

The Obesity Epidemic

More than 2 in 3 adults are considered to be overweight or have obesity in the United States. In other words, being overweight or obese is the new normal for Americans.

Unfortunately, carrying more than a few extra pounds is an epidemic throughout the world as well. Since 1975, the prevalence of obesity in the global population has tripled. Now, more than 1.9 billion adults aged 18 years and older are overweight. Of these adults, over 650 million are obese.

Each one of these people carries an increased risk of cardiovascular disease, musculoskeletal disorders (e.g., arthritis and low back pain), cancer, type 2 diabetes, and depression. What's even more frightening is that as the weight continues to increase so does the risk for this noncommunicable diseases.

And yet, despite how obvious it is that being obese is unhealthy, obesity rates are still climbing. Simply telling people to eat less and move more isn't enough — one of the primary causes of this issue runs much deeper than self-control.

The Potential Causes of The Obesity Epidemic

Just like most health issues, many different factors contribute to obesity. The factors most responsible for the obesity epidemic seem to be our genetics and the environment, and how they interact to create our eating behavior. To gain a deeper understanding of how they contribute to obesity, let's explore the organ responsible for our eating decisions the brain.

The brain was built over millions of years of genetic evolution. The evolution of the brain (and its deeply ingrained behavioral patterns) depended on its ability to adapt to an environment that shared almost nothing in common with where we spend most of our time today.

The first humans didn't have Walmart, grocery stores, and restaurants around every corner they had wild plants to forage and animals to hunt that may or may, not be there the next day. To adapt to this uncertain food environment, humans and all other animals developed a highly motivating and rewarding relationship with food.

As a result, humans and most other animals tend to eat much more than necessary in an attempt to store extra calories and other nutrients away for times when food is scarce. To put it more simply, we are wired to eat as much as possible when food is available.

More specifically, we are wired to seek out foods that contain different combinations of fat, carbs, protein, and salt. More food variety means more nutrients and better survival.

Given the choice of a fat and protein source like meat or a salt and carb rich food like potato chips, we are designed say yes to both. No matter how stuffed we are, the most primal parts of our brain will typically tell us that there is room for more if a novel food source is available. These behaviors were essential for our survival as a species. If we ate reasonably whenever food was available, then we wouldn't have enough fat or muscle to fuel us when calories were scarce.

Unfortunately, our current food environment is nothing like what the human race initially evolved to handle. Today, we are constantly bombarded with endless processed food options, food ads, and smells that trigger our desires. As a result, the oldest parts of our brain motivate us to hunt for that food, which we now have a 100% chance of getting and we don't have to exert much effort at all to get it.

We will then act out our ancestral programming by eating the most calorie dense foods (i.e., pizza, french fries, cookies, cakes, etc.) and eating much more of those foods then what our body needs to energize itself until the next meal. This results in a vicious cycle of overeating and weight gain with the subconscious intention to prepare us for famine famine that never comes.

When we consider our genetics and the current food environment together, a fascinating story reveals itself. The human species evolved from millions of years of genes that were trying to survive an environment that they didn't create. As a result, humans evolved the ability to create their own environment that allows them to fulfill their needs at any given moment with minimal effort.

The irony in all of this is that the very genes that provided us with this astounding ability to create our own food environment have not been given enough time to adapt to the abundance that the majority of the human species created for themselves.

The result? A profound mismatch between the human and its environment that causes it to eat so much and move so little that humanity accelerates its own extinction. For a more specific example, take another look at how many people are obese or overweight in the United States a country with one of the most convenient food environments.

The solution? One way of approaching this issue is through dieting. To adapt to such an abundant food environment, you need to give your brain new food rules to follow (e.g, a diet). Your brain needs you to tell it what to eat and what not to eat to meet your health goals. One of the best ways to do this is by finding a diet with simple rules that you can follow for the rest of your life.

The Best Diet For Weight Loss

Health is so complex that there is no "best diet for weight loss." Every person requires unique dietary and lifestyle changes so that they can lose weight and keep it off for the rest of their life.

What we do know for certain is that calories matter. (The human body cannot escape the laws of thermodynamics.) If you eat more than your body needs to maintain itself, then you will gain weight. Conversely, if you eat less than your body needs, then you will lose weight. It's a simple concept, but it comes with a ton of nuances.

Your daily caloric needs are not set in stone they vary slightly from day to day. Because of the unpredictable nature of our calorie requirements, many scientists have posited that they don't matter as much as other things like hormones.

The carbohydrate-insulin hypothesis, for example, proposes that the primary cause of the obesity epidemic is insulin stimulating foods like sugar and starches. The logic behind this hypothesis is based on one of the many actions of insulin.

When carbs are consumed, insulin is released by the pancreas. Once insulin interacts with fat cells, it prevents fat from being burned as fuel and triggers fat storage.

Because of this phenomenon, the supporters of the carbohydrate-insulin hypothesis tend to believe that all you need to do to lose fat is restrict carbs. However, this is a reductionistic view of obesity that doesn't account for the complex nature of the human body.

The truth is that there are multiple mechanisms for fat storage in the body that depend on calorie intake, not insulin. Insulin has also been shown to play a role in regulating our metabolic rate, which increases our caloric output to a minimal degree.

To sum up what we learned in this section, here's a helpful way to think of weight loss: Calorie intake makes the biggest impact on whether you gain or lose weight.

Other factors like exercise and insulin also matter, but to a much smaller degree.

The current literature argues between calories and carbohydrates. Below, we discuss it further.

Calories or Carbs?

Instead of focusing on switching out carbs for fat or vice versa, we should focus on sticking to a diet that naturally decreases our calorie intake.

How can we naturally decrease our calorie intake? The two most effective ways are:

Eating a diet that consists of protein-dense and fiber-rich foods because of how satiating they are.

Eliminating all calorically-dense processed foods from your diet because of how easy it is to binge on them.

One of the diets that implement this principles is the low-carb ketogenic diet. It primarily consists of highly-satiating foods like meat and low-carb vegetables while cutting out all carb-ridden, highly-palatable foods. By eating in this way, most people experience tremendous amounts of fat loss not because it lowers insulin levels, but because keto dieters tend to eat significantly fewer calories than high-carb dieters without realizing it.

Low-fat or Keto?

The meta-analysis provide us with very convincing data, but we must also consider the fact that the data came from studies where all the food was provided by the scientists. Although this is a great way to assess the difference between low-carb and high-carb diet, this does not simulate the real-world effectiveness of each diet. For this reason, we must investigate data from less strict studies. In other words, we need to look at what happened when subjects were told to follow a specific diet on their own.

They specifically looked at trials that compared a ketogenic diet that consisted of no more than 50 grams of carbs per day with a conventional, low-fat diet with less than 30% of calories from fat.

When examining the results, the researchers found that the participants in the ketogenic diet groups lost an average of 2 more pounds than the low-fat diet groups. The researchers also noted greater improvements in triglycerides, blood pressure, and HDL cholesterol in the ketogenic diet groups.

As a result, the researchers concluded that the ketogenic diet "may be an alternative tool against obesity."

These findings fall in line with another meta-analysis on 13 randomized controlled trials that compared low-fat and low-carbohydrate diets. The researchers found that, after six months, subjects who consumed less than 60 grams of carbohydrates per day had an average weight loss that was 8.8 pounds greater than the subjects on low-fat diets. At one year, the difference had fallen to 2.3 lb (which is consistent with what was found in the meta-analysis conducted by the Brazilian researchers).

As a result, the researchers concluded that "low-carbohydrate/high-protein diets are more effective at 6 months and are as effective, if not more, as low-fat diets in reducing weight and cardiovascular disease risk up to 1 year."

These two meta-analyses (and the other research you'll find in this article on keto & weight loss) provide us with a look at the real world significance of low-fat and low-carb diets. When you put people on a low-carb ketogenic type diet, they tend to lose more weight than people who are on a low-fat diet. The ketogenic diet also provides us with clear rules to follow, which makes it is easier for us to keep ourselves from overeating.

To put it another way, the ketogenic diet is one of the best ways to "hack" our brain and food environment so that we naturally eat fewer calories and lose weight. What is even more interesting is that this isn't the only reason why many people find weight loss success with keto.

Ketosis for Weight Loss

When carbohydrates are restricted for a couple of days, the body will start to produce ketones. This alternative fuel source comes with many benefits for the brain and nervous system, while it simultaneously promotes weight loss.

Once the body enters ketosis and starts to burn ketones for fuel, most ketogenic dieters will experience increased energy levels and decreased appetite. This leads to the consumption of fewer calories, resulting in more weight loss.

Another reason why ketosis and weight loss are linked is that ketones have a mild diuretic effect. This is important to know because many people will mistake their rapid weight loss on keto as if it is all coming from fat. In reality, the rapid weight loss that occurs in the first week of the ketogenic diet is mostly due to water loss.

Rapid Weight Loss on the Ketogenic Diet

Typically, during the first week of the keto diet, people see a very quick drop in weight — anywhere from 2 to 10 pounds. This is unrivaled by any other diet, but it is also not all coming from fat.

In fact, most of this weight loss is the result of the body shedding the extra water weight it was holding on to as a consequence of carbohydrate consumption. This can cause flu- like symptoms, which is why it is essential to drink plenty of water and follow the suggestions that you'll find in our guide to the keto flu.

After a week or two of keto dieting, weight loss will happen at a slower and more steady pace. This is also the period of time when the body becomes keto-adapted as it switches from burning carbs to burning fat.

How Fast Will You Lose Weight with Keto?

Once you've made it through the first week of keto and you are in ketosis, fat will steadily fall off your body (as long as you are in a calorie deficit). The average weight loss at this point is around 1-2 pounds per week the majority of it coming from fat.

As you get closer to your goal weight and your overall body weight decreases, weight loss will slow down. This happens because as your weight decreases so will your daily caloric needs. For this reason, you may want to recalculate your calorie needs every month or so.

Keep in mind that weight loss may, not be consistent either. You might have some weeks where it seems you haven't lost anything then you'll weigh yourself a week or two later and be down 3-4 pounds.

How Fast Will You Lose Weight with Keto?

What is behind the seemingly unpredictable and unique nature of your weight loss rate? Here are some of the critical factors that determine how fast the pounds will come off:

Your calorie deficit. The one factor that leads to the most significant and consistent weight loss is a calorie deficit. In other words, when we consume fewer calories than we need to maintain our weight, we will lose weight. This means that your weight loss rate will usually increase as your total calorie consumption decreases. However, there are limits to how far you should take you should take your deficit. The human body is designed to prevent massive amounts of weight loss during times of starvation via mechanisms that make long-term fat loss much harder to achieve and maintain. Because of this, it is never a good idea to starve yourself for extended periods of time. Research indicates that calorie deficits above 30% are enough to stimulate some of these counterproductive mechanisms for long-term fat loss.

Your current health status. Your overall health plays a major role in how fast you will lose weight and adapt to a lower carb diet. If you have any hormonal or metabolic issues, weight loss might be slower or a bit more challenging than expected. Insulin resistance, excess visceral fat, and thyroid issues, for example, can all have a significant impact on your weight loss rate.

Your body composition. Do you have a lot of fat to lose? How much muscle do you have? The people who have the most to lose will tend to shred the fat at a much faster rate than those who have a few extra pounds to burn off. This phenomenon is mostly explained by the fact that obese individuals can easily maintain a much larger calorie deficit, which will result in faster weight loss. Muscle mass also plays a vital role in weight loss because it helps keep your metabolic rate from dropping significantly as you lose weight. This can help stabilize your weight loss rate and may even prevent a dreaded weight loss plateau.

Your daily habits. Your daily habits will make or break your weight loss efforts. Consistency is the key to keto success. Are you eating clean keto foods or high-fat junk foods with low-quality ingredients? Are you watching out for hidden carbs? Are you exercising? Eating the right foods in the right amounts for your goals and adding more physical activity to your daily life is the most important pieces of a smooth and successful body transformation.

When we take a step back and look at the bigger picture of our fat loss rate, predictable patterns began to emerge. For example, the people who typically see the slowest weight loss are those who are sedentary and overweight with poor metabolic health and eating habits that don't exercise or keep track of their carb and/or calorie consumption.

Conversely, those who start with more muscle and decent metabolic health that are disciplined enough to stick to their diet plan, maintain a calorie deficit, and increase their physical activity levels will typically lose weight more quickly and get the results they want.

In general, everyone's health and lifestyle is different, which means the weight loss rate for each person is going to be different too. We do, however, share one thing in common: each one of us can optimize our body composition with our diets.

How Much Weight Loss Will You Get from Following the Keto Diet?

With a well-formulated keto diet, you can technically drop as much fat as you want.

Yes, you read that correctly – you have the potential to sculpt your body into incredible shape with keto. However, most of us will not reach our body composition goals by simple restricting carbs and being in ketosis.

From a dietary perspective, getting the results that you desire will take discipline, consistency, and a well-formulated, healthy dietary approach. The discipline and consistency are up to you; our job is to provide you with the information that will help you reach your goals with the keto diet.

To help you get started on your weight loss journey, we put together a list of the four fundamental principles that will help you formulate a healthy keto diet for your needs:

Eat the right amount of calories and protein to meet your goals. You can use our keto calculator and calorie tracking guide to help you with this.

Get most of your calories from micronutrient dense foods. For more detailed information on what to eat, check out our guide to micronutrients and our keto food list.

Make sure your diet is improving your overall health and wellbeing subjectively and objectively.

Implement lifestyle adjustments to make your diet into a long-term lifestyle that you can follow indefinitely.

You will know that you are following a well-formulated and healthy keto diet for you if these four variables are trending in the right direction:

Your mood, energy levels, and sense of well-being Your

body composition

Relevant biomarkers (e.g., blood pressure, cholesterol, triglyceride, and blood sugar levels)

Your ketone levels

For more information on how to create a keto diet that is healthy and effective for you, we recommend checking out our recent article on the topic.

However, even if you follow every suggestion and strategy flawlessly, you may end up stalling at the same weight for a few weeks. In this case, you may need to make some minor adjustments to your diet to get back on track.

How to Break Through Plateaus and Boost Weight Loss on the Ketogenic Diet

Plateaus are an inevitable part of every diet. Eventually, you will get to a point where you are eating what your body needs to maintain its weight. This can happen months to years after you start the keto diet.

When you encounter the dreaded plateau, don't give up simply follow some of these suggestions:

Track your calories. If you are not already doing so, track your calories using an app like Cronometer. This simple habit will take your results to the next level because you'll have an objective way of knowing if you are eating the right amount of carbs, fat, protein, and calories every day.

Recalculate your macronutrient targets. When you hit a plateau or simply want to boost your fat loss, plug your updated information into the keto calculator. This will allow you to maintain a calorie deficit even after your calorie needs have dropped.

Experiment with fat fasting. If you are still struggling, try implementing a technique called the fat fast. It normally consists of a three-day window of low caloric intake and high amounts of fat to kickstart fat burning and increase fat loss. If you're interested, I went into more detail on fat fasting in another post.

Eat less often. It's much easier to eat fewer calories and maintain higher levels of ketosis when you eat less meals. Instead of snacking throughout the day, try getting all of your calories from 2-3 meals every day. You can also try intermittent fasting by restricting all your meals to an 8-hour eating window. This will allow your blood sugar and insulin to drop down to baseline levels so that your body can go into its fasting state and burn body fat for fuel.

Stick to the ketogenic diet (no cheating). Going from keto to high-carb will cause you to gain weight rapidly. Even just one cheat day can cause you to gain 4 to 6 pounds of water weight. If you have a sugar craving, indulge in a keto-friendly dessert instead of a sugar-filled snack.

Don't eat foods that you are sensitive to. If your body struggles with dairy, gluten, or other foods in any way, then consider eliminating it from your diet. Food sensitivities can slow progress and impair health.

Check for hidden carb sources. You may be eating more carbs than you think. Make sure you aren't getting too many carbs from sneaky sources like vegetables, peanut butter, processed meats, and over-the-counter medications.

Decrease your stress levels. The most common ways that people stress their bodies on a diet is by eating too little and exercising too much. Studies have found that exercising for more than an hour a day can drop our metabolic rate by 15%, and maintaining a caloric deficit of 25% can decrease our metabolic rate by 6%. In other words, don't overdo it you will slow your metabolism down and cause your own weight loss plateau.

Eat the right amount of protein. Too much protein can increase insulin levels and decrease ketone levels, while not consuming enough protein can cause you to burn muscle rather than fat. If you exercise, protein levels should be hovering around 0.8g – 1.0g protein per lean pound of body mass a day. This helps with muscle mass retention and growth. However, if you are not exercising – your protein intake doesn't need to be as high. A protein intake of 0.6g – 0.8g of protein per lean pound of body mass is going to be fine for sedentary individuals.

Lift weights. By lifting weights, you will build muscle mass and modestly increase your metabolic rate and fat loss. One of the best ways to increase muscle mass is by doing bodybuilding type workouts. For an overview of how to gain muscle on keto, check out our guide to keto bodybuilding.

Take calorie deficit breaks. If nothing else seems to work, then try taking intermittent diet breaks every two weeks or so. Recent research found that obese men who took 2 week breaks from being in a caloric deficit lost more fat than the men who maintained a calorie deficit. This means that keto dieters may benefit from taking intermittent calorie deficit breaks as well. To implement a diet break, simply follow the ketogenic diet for two weeks while you maintain a calorie deficit. After that two weeks, calculate what you need to eat to maintain your bodyweight, aim to eat that many calories, and repeat recalculating your calorie deficit after each calorie maintenance phase. Researchers hypothesize that this method of dieting helps keep your metabolism from slowing down, allowing you to burn more calories while you are in a calorie deficit.

Looking for more specific info on how to bust through weight loss plateaus on the ketogenic diet? Follow this link to learn more.

However, there is one caveat when it comes to weight loss. In response to a calorie deficit, the body will typically burn some of its muscle mass for fuel by using a process called gluconeogenesis. As a result, many people will lose muscle along with the fat when they diet. Luckily, there is a way to preserve muscle mass, even in the midst of extreme caloric deficits.

How To Avoid Muscle Loss On Keto

The most important macronutrient for preserving and building lean muscle is protein. Carbs help preserve muscle mass to some extent, but protein is — without a doubt — the most important macronutrient that you must eat enough if you don't want to lose muscle.

Protein consumption is especially crucial on the ketogenic diet. Without dietary carbs to provoke an anabolic (muscle building) response, you will tend to lose muscle more rapidly without adequate protein intake on keto.

With that being said, research has also found that ketones have a muscle preserving effect. Because of this, it is reasonable to suggest that you should eat just enough protein to maintain muscle mass without eating so much protein that you decrease your ketone levels.

How To Avoid Muscle Loss On Keto

Here is the protein intake that we recommend for keto dieters:

If you exercise, protein levels should be hovering around 0.8g – 1.0g protein per lean pound of body mass a day.

If you are sedentary, then your protein intake should be between 0.6g – 0.8g per lean pound of body mass.

The higher the caloric deficit, the closer your protein intake should be to the higher end of the range.

Keep in mind, however, that consuming too much protein at any given meal can decrease your levels of ketosis. To mitigate this effect, you can divide your protein intake into equal amounts throughout your meals. If you workout, then consider consuming more protein after and/or before your workouts because this protein is less likely to spike insulin levels and reduce ketone levels.

However, even if you follow all the recommendations in this article, you still won't know for certain if you are actually losing fat. To get a more accurate measure of your fat loss, it is essential to estimate and track your body fat percentage.

How to Track Your Fat Loss on the Ketogenic Diet

There are many methods you can use to evaluate your fat loss, but the two simplest ways are by visually estimating your body fat percentage and by plugging your waist circumference, height, and weight into a body fat calculator.

On the other hand, if you'd like to use a body fat calculator, here's what you do: Wrap the tape measure around your waist at the level of your belly button.

Exhale all your air and secure the tape without stretching it.

Read the measurement, write it down, and calculate your percentage of body fat by plugging it into this body fat calculator.

Remeasure every 2 to 4 weeks to track your progress.

How to Track Your Fat Loss on the Ketogenic Diet

Although this isn't particularly accurate, it will provide you with a reasonable estimate of your body fat % that you can track while you are dieting. You can also look at your body fat % estimate along with your weight and waist circumference to determine if the weight you lost is fat or water.

Waist circumference, for example, tends to decrease as fat mass decreases, providing you with an indicator that you lost fat. If your goal is to gain muscle mass and lose fat, then the numbers on the scale should either increase or stay the same as the numbers on the measuring tape and your body fat % calculation decrease.

Losing Weight on Keto

The bulk of research suggests that the ketogenic diet is more effective than conventional diets in helping you lose weight and shed body fat. One of the reasons why the ketogenic diet provides such reliable weight loss results is because it consists primarily of highly- satiating whole foods like meat, high-fat dairy, and low-carb vegetables while removing all carb-rich, sugar-laden processed foods from the diet. By eating in this way, you will feel full while eating fewer calories and losing weight.

The most important part of the ketogenic diet is consistency. Approach this diet (or any other diet that you try) with the mindset that you will make it into a long-term sustainable lifestyle. When you hit a plateau, don't give up we all hit plateaus eventually. Take it as an opportunity to recalculate your calorie needs, adjust your goals, and implement new strategies.

To maximize your fat loss on keto even further, follow these suggestions: Track your macronutrient consumption

Aim to reduce your waist circumference and body fat % Eat the right amount of protein

Reduce your stress levels Lift weights

Supplement your diet with MCTs and CLA

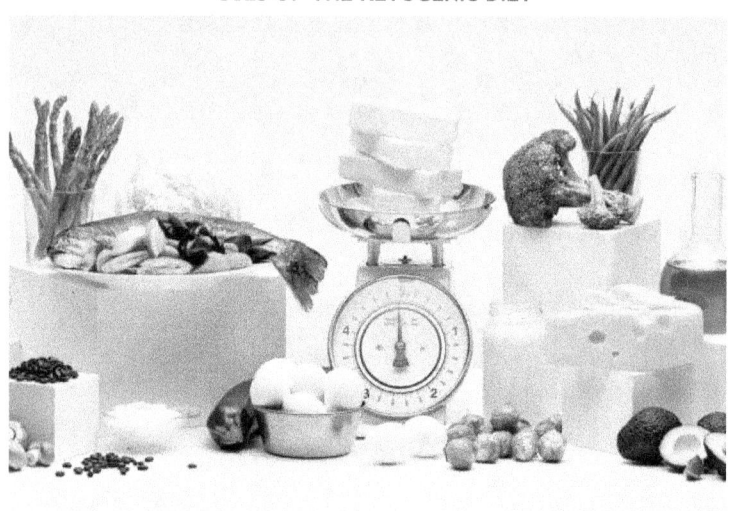

When using a ketogenic diet, your body becomes more of a fat-burner than a carbohydrate-dependent machine. Several researches have linked the consumption of increased amounts of carbohydrates to development of several disorders such as diabetes and insulin resistance.

By nature, carbohydrates are easily absorbable and therefore can be also be easily stored by the body. Digestion of carbohydrates starts right from the moment you put them into your mouth.

As soon as you begin chewing them, amylase (the enzymes that digest carbohydrate) in your saliva is already at work acting on the carbohydrate-containing food.

In the stomach, carbohydrates are further broken down. When they get into the small intestines, they are then absorbed into the bloodstream. On getting to the bloodstream, carbohydrates generally increase the blood sugar level.

This increase in blood sugar level stimulates the immediate release of insulin into the bloodstream. The higher the increase in blood sugar levels, the more the amount of insulin that is release.

Insulin is a hormone that causes excess sugar in the bloodstream to be removed in order to lower the blood sugar level. Insulin takes the sugar and carbohydrate that you eat and stores them either as glycogen in muscle tissues or as fat in adipose tissue for future use as energy.

However, the body can develop what is known as insulin resistance when it is continuously exposed to such high amounts of glucose in the bloodstream. This scenario can easily cause obesity as the body tends to quickly store any excess amount of glucose. Health conditions such as diabetes and cardiovascular disease can also result from this condition.

Keto diets are low in carbohydrate and high in fat and have been associated with reducing and improving several health conditions.

One of the foremost things a ketogenic diet does is to stabilize your insulin levels and also restore leptin signalling. Reduced amounts of insulin in the bloodstream allow you to feel fuller for a longer period of time and also to have fewer cravings.

Medical Benefits of Ketogenic Diets

The application and implementation of the ketogenic diet has expanded considerably. Keto diets are often indicated as part of the treatment plan in a number of medical conditions.

Epilepsy

This is basically the main reason for the development of the ketogenic diet. For some reason, the rate of epileptic seizures reduces when patients are placed on a keto diet.

Pediatric epileptic cases are the most responsive to the keto diet. There are children who have experience seizure elimination after a few years of using a keto diet.

Children with epilepsy is generally expected to fast for a few days before starting the ketogenic diet as part of their treatment.

Cancer

Research suggests that the therapeutic efficacy of the ketogenic diets against tumor growth can be enhanced when combined with certain drugs and procedures under a "press-pulse" paradigm.

It is also promising to note that ketogenic diets drive the cancer cell into remission. This means that keto diets "starves cancer" to reduce the symptoms.

Alzheimer Disease

There are several indications that the memory functions of patients with Alzheimer's disease improve after making use of a ketogenic diet.

Ketones are a great source of alternative energy for the brain especially when it has become resistant to insulin. Ketones also provide substrates (cholesterol) that help to repair damaged neurons and membranes. These all help to improve memory and cognition in Alzheimer patients.

Diabetes

It is generally agreed that carbohydrates are the main culprit in diabetes. Therefore, by reducing the amount of ingested carbohydrate by using a ketogenic diet, there are increased chances for improved blood sugar control.

Also, combining a keto diet with other diabetes treatment plans can significantly improve their overall effectiveness.

Gluten Allergy

Many individuals with gluten allergy are undiagnosed with this condition. However, following a ketogenic diet showed improvement in related symptoms like digestive discomforts and bloating.

Most carbohydrate-rich foods are high in gluten. Thus, by using a keto diet, a lot of the gluten consumption is reduced to a minimum due to the elimination of a large variety of carbohydrates.

Weight Loss

This is arguably the most common "intentional" use of the ketogenic diet today. It has found a niche for itself in the mainstream dieting trend. Keto diets have become part of many dieting regimen due to its well acknowledged side effect of aiding weight loss.

Though initially maligned by many, the growing number of favorable weight loss results has helped the ketogenic to better embraced as a major weight loss program.

Besides the above medical benefits, ketogenic diets also provide some general health benefits which include the following.

Improved Insulin Sensitivity

This is obviously the first aim of a ketogenic diet. It helps to stabilize your insulin levels thereby improving fat burning.

Muscle Preservation

Since protein is oxidized, it helps to preserve lean muscle. Losing lean muscle mass causes an individual's metabolism to slow down as muscles are generally very metabolic. Using a keto diet actually helps to preserve your muscles while your body burns fat.

Controlled pH and respiratory function

A ketoc diet helps to decrease lactate thereby improving both pH and respiratory function. A state of ketosis therefore helps to keep your blood pH at a healthy level.

Improved Immune System

Using a ketogenic diet helps to fight off aging antioxidants while also reducing inflammation of the gut thereby making your immune system stronger.

Reduced Cholesterol Levels

Consuming fewer carbohydrates while you are on the keto diet will help to reduce blood cholesterol levels. This is due to the increased state of lipolysis. This leads to a reduction in LDL cholesterol levels and an increase in HDL cholesterol levels.

Reduced Appetite and Cravings

Adopting a ketogenic diet helps you to reduce both your appetite and cravings for calorie rich foods. As you begin eating healthy, satisfying, and beneficial high-fat foods, your hunger feelings will naturally start decreasing.

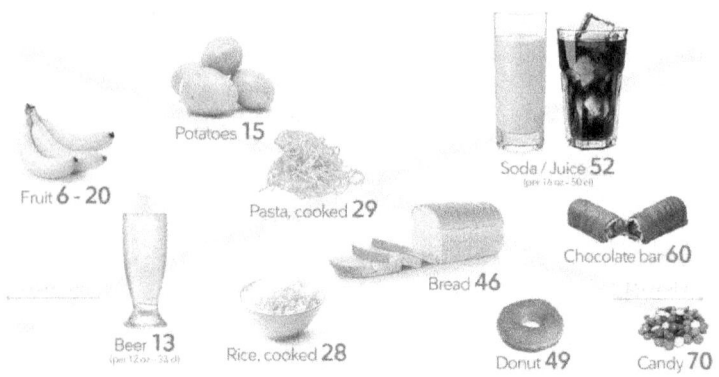

Potatoes 15

Soda / Juice 52
(per 16 oz - 50 cl)

Fruit 6 - 20

Pasta, cooked 29

Chocolate bar 60

Bread 46

Beer 13
(per 12 oz - 33 cl)

Rice, cooked 28

Donut 49

Candy 70

A ketogenic diet is basically a diet which converts your body from burning sugar to burning fat. Around 99% of the wold's population have a diet which cause their body to burn sugar. As a result, carbohydrates are their primary fuel source used after digesting carbs. This process makes people gain weight, however a diet of fat and ketones will cause weight loss. As you ask what can you eat on a ketogenic diet, first of all eat up to 30 to 50 grams of carbs per day. Next, let us discover more about what you can have on your plate and how the ketogenic diet affects your health.

The Importance Of Sugar Precaution On The Ketogenic Diet

Keto shifts your body from a sugar burner to a fat burner by eliminating the dietary sugar derived from carbohydrates. The first obvious reduction you should make from your current diet is sugar and sugary foods. Although sugar is a definite target for deletion, the ketogenic diet focuses upon the limitation of carbohydrates. We need to watch out for sugar in a number of different types of foods and nutrients. Even a white potato which is carb-heavy may not taste sweet to your tongue like sugar. But once it hits your bloodstream after digestion, those carbs add the simple sugar known as glucose to your body. The truth is, our body can only store so much glucose before it dumps it elsewhere in our system. Excess glucose becomes what is known as the fat which accumulates in our stomach region, love handles, etc.

Protein And It's Place In Keto

One source of carbohydrates which some people overlook in their diet is protein. Overconsumption of protein according to the tolerance level of your body will result in weight gain. Because our body converts excess protein into sugar, we must moderate the amount of protein we eat. Moderation of our protein intake is part of how to eat ketogenic and lose weight. First of all, identify your own tolerance of daily protein and use as a guide to maintain an optimal intake of the nutrient. Second, choose your protein from foods such as organic cage-free eggs and grass-fed meats. Finally, create meals in variety that are delicious and maintain your interest in the diet. For instance, a 5 ounce steak and a few eggs can provide an ideal amount of daily protein for some people.

Caloric Intake On The Ketogenic Diet

Calories are another important consideration for what can you eat on a ketogenic diet. Energy derived from the calories in the food we consume help our body to remain functional. Hence, we must eat enough calories in order to meet our daily nutritional requirements. Counting calories is a burden for many people who are on other diets. But as a ketogenic dieter, you don't have to worry nearly as much about calorie counting. Most people on a low-carb diet remain satisfied by eating a daily amount of 1500-1700 kcals in calories.

Fats, The Good & The Bad

Fat is not bad, in fact many good healthy fats exist in whole foods such as nuts, seeds and olive oil. Healthy fats are an integral part of the ketogenic diet and are available as spreads, snacks and toppings. Misconceptions in regards to eating fat are that a high amount of it is unhealthy and causes weight gain. While both statements are in a sense true, the fat which we consume is not the direct cause of the fat which appears on our body. Rather, the sugar from each nutrient we consume is what eventually becomes the fat on our body.

Balance Your Nutrients Wisely

Digestion causes the sugars we eat to absorb into the bloodstream and the excess amount transfer into our fat cells. High carbohydrate and high protein eating will result in excess body fat, because there is sugar content in these nutrients. So excessive eating of any nutrient is unhealthy and causes weight gain. But a healthy diet consists of a balance of protein, carbohydrates and fats according to the tolerance levels of your body.

Just about everyone can accomplish a ketogenic diet with enough persistence and effort. In addition, we can moderate a number of bodily conditions naturally with keto. Insulin resistance, elevated blood sugar, inflammation, obesity, type-2 diabetes are some health conditions that keto can help to stabilize. Each of these unhealthy conditions will reduce and normalize for the victim who follows a healthy ketogenic diet. Low-carb, high-fat and moderate protein whole foods provide the life-changing health benefits of this diet.

WHAT ARE THE SIGNS OF KETOSIS

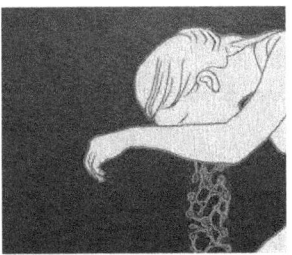

Ketosis is a metabolic process that occurs when the body begins to burn fat for energy because it does not have enough carbohydrates to burn. During this process, the liver produces chemicals called ketones.

The ketogenic, or keto, diet aims to induce ketosis in order to burn more fat. Proponents of the diet claim that it boosts weight loss and improves overall health.

Despite these guidelines, some people following the diet may not know when they are in ketosis.

we list 10 signs and symptoms that may help a person determine whether the ketogenic diet is working for them.

1 Increased ketones

A blood sample can indicate ketone levels.

Having ketones in the blood is probably the most definitive sign that someone is in ketosis. Doctors may also use urine and breath tests to check for ketone levels, but these are less reliable than blood samples.

A special home testing kit allows people to measure their own blood ketone levels. Or, a doctor may take a blood sample and send it away for testing. When a person is in nutritional ketosis, they will have blood ketone levels of 0.5–3 millimoles per liter.

Alternatively, people can use a breath analyzer to test for ketones in their breath, or they may use indicator strips to check their urinary levels.

2 Weight loss

Some research suggests that this type of very-low-carbohydrate diet is effective for weight loss. Therefore, people should expect to lose some weight when in ketosis.

The results of 2013 meta-analysis that examined the findings from several randomized controlled trials suggest that people following a ketogenic diet may lose more weight in the long-term than people following a low-fat diet.

People on a ketogenic diet may notice weight loss in the first few days, but this is typically just a reduction in water weight. True fat loss may not occur for several weeks.

3 Thirst

Ketosis may cause some people to feel thirstier than usual, which may occur as a side effect of water loss. However, high levels of ketones in the body can also lead to dehydration and an electrolyte imbalance. Both of these reactions can cause complications.

Research into ketogenic diets for sports performance lists dehydration as a side effect of ketosis. Athletes may also have a higher risk of kidney stones, which is a complication of dehydration.

To avoid dehydration, drink plenty of water and other liquids. See a doctor if symptoms of dehydration, such as extreme thirst or dark-colored urine, occur.

4 Muscle cramps and spasms

Dehydration and electrolyte imbalances can cause muscle cramps. Electrolytes are substances that carry electrical signals between the body's cells. Imbalances in these substances lead to disrupted electrical messages that may cause muscle contractions and spasms.

People following the ketogenic diet should ensure that they are getting enough electrolytes from the food they eat to avoid muscle pains and other symptoms of an imbalance.

Electrolytes include calcium, magnesium, potassium, and sodium. A person can get these from eating a balanced diet. However, if symptoms persist, a doctor may recommend supplements or other dietary changes.

5 Headaches

Ketosis headaches can last from 1 to 7 days, or longer.

Headaches can be a common side effect of switching to a ketogenic diet. They may occur as a result of consuming fewer carbohydrates, especially sugar. Dehydration and electrolyte imbalances can also cause headaches.

Ketosis headaches typically last from 1 day to 1 week, although some people may experience pain for longer. See a doctor if headaches persist.

6 Fatigue and weakness

In the initial stages of a ketosis diet, people may feel more tired and weaker than usual. This fatigue occurs as the body switches from burning carbohydrates to burning fat for energy. Carbohydrates provide a quicker burst of energy to the body.

A small 2017 study involving athletes found tiredness to be a common side effect of the ketosis diet. Participants typically observed this during the first few weeks.

After several weeks on the diet, people should notice an increase in their energy levels. If not, they should seek medical attention, as fatigue is also a symptom of dehydration and nutrient deficiencies.

7 Stomach complaints

Making any dietary changes can raise the risk of stomach upset and other digestive complaints. This may also occur when a person switches to the ketogenic diet.

To reduce the risk of experiencing stomach complaints, drink plenty of water and other fluids. Eat non-starchy vegetables and other fiber-rich foods to alleviate constipation, and consider taking a probiotic supplement to encourage a healthy gut.

8 Changes in sleep

Following a ketogenic diet may disrupt a person's sleeping habits. Initially, they may experience difficulty falling asleep or nighttime waking. These symptoms typically go away within a few weeks.

9 Bad breath

A common side effect of ketosis is bad breath.

Bad breath is among the most common side effects of ketosis. This is because ketones leave the body through the breath as well as the urine. People on the diet, or those around them, may notice that the breath smells sweet or fruity.

A ketone called acetone is usually responsible for the odor, but other ketones, such as benzophenone and acetophenone, may also contribute to bad breath.

There is no way to reduce ketosis breath, but it may improve with time. Some people use sugar-free gum or brush their teeth several times per day to mask the smell.

10 Better focus and concentration

Initially, the ketogenic diet may cause headaches and concentration difficulties. However, these symptoms should fade over time. People following a long-term ketogenic diet often report better clarity and focus, and some research supports this.

According to the results of a 2018 systematic review, people with epilepsy who follow the ketogenic diet report better alertness and attention. Also, these people showed greater alertness in some cognitive tests.

A KETOGENIC DIET FOR PHYSICAL PERFORMANCE

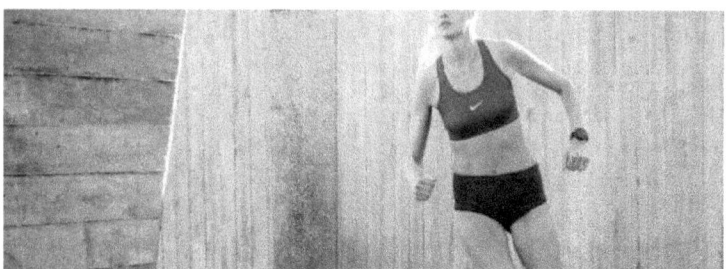

Should those who are physically active continue eating low-carb? It's a fair question for those wanting to follow a ketogenic diet for better health, and that's why we'll be exploring the main areas of ketosis for physical performance.

The ketogenic diet and ketosis have been used traditionally by physicians and other professionals for a few different medical reasons, including improving the health of those with diabetes and treating neurological disorders like epilepsy.

But now, we've begun to explore other factors where the ketogenic diet can have a positive effect, including mental focus, weight loss, and in this article, ketosis for physical performance.

The Ketogenic Diet for Exercise

While the emphasis for exercise is usually on high carbohydrate intake, the ketogenic diet takes a low-carb approach to energy. Those on a ketogenic diet generally stay within a range of 30-50 grams of carbs per day, and a large amount of food in the diet comes from fat.

The ketogenic diet involves a dietary breakdown of: Low

carbohydrate intake

Moderate protein intake High

fat intake

The low intake of carbs is meant to put the dieter into ketosis, where the body creates ketones from fat stores to use as the main energy source, instead of carbs, for the body and even partly for the brain. Molecules known as ketones are produced during the process.

This means that someone exercising while eating a ketogenic diet is going to be using primarily fat as fuel for their physical activity.

Misconceptions About Ketosis For Physical Performance

A long-held belief among the nutrition and medical community is that carbohydrates must make up a high portion of your diet in order to maintain physical performance at an ideal level. This belief mostly stems from studies in the last 100 years looking at muscle glycogen and its link to high intensity exercise.

However, there are few reasons to question this thought process:

We've observed cultures that didn't eat in line with the carb-heavy philosophy, such as the Inuit people in the Canadian and Alaskan Arctic regions. Before their diets changed a lot, scientists were able to observe their traditional diet and see that it contained virtually no known carbohydrates, yet they were able to function normally physically.

Demographic evidence of past European cultures has shown them living as primarily hunters without any noted physical impediments.

While diets with more carbohydrates may prove better for higher-intensity, short-term forms of exercise, the limitations of the ketogenic diet for physical performance have been over exaggerated. In fact, ketosis can have a healthy role in relation physical activity for most individuals.

Let's take a look at the differences associated with using ketones for fuel versus using carbs for fuel.

Fat Adaptation In Ketosis

With a ketogenic or other low carb diet, the body experiences fat adaptation, or keto- adaption, where it becomes more efficient at burning fat and ketones for fuel. This adaptation can be strong and have a great impact on the fat burning process during exercise.

During a recent study, ultra-endurance athletes who were on a ketogenic diet for an average of 20 months were shown to burn up to 2.3 times more fat than the high-carb group during a three-hour run. The study also found that muscle glycogen use and repletion during and after the exercise was similar between the low-carb and high-carb groups. This is a significant demonstration of the power of keto-adaptation for exercise.

Endurance Exercise And Ketosis

As we've established, fat can be used for energy when carbs aren't available for use. While carbs do provide more fuel for the body to perform at higher intensities, fat is what provides more energy during exercise at lower intensities.

However, this might be open to question as well. In one study, researchers recorded athletes following a ketogenic diet had burned mostly fat during exercise at up to 70% of their max intensity, while the high-carb athletes burned fat at 55%. This again demonstrates the increased effectiveness of ketosis for fuel during exercise when a person's body has adapted to burning primarily fat for energy.

With this in mind, it's still important to recognize that some elite athletes may require energy more quickly than the rate at which they can get it from fat, and more research is needed on the subject to know the details for sure.

That being said, a low-carb ketogenic diet can be helpful in regards to exercise for:

Preventing tiredness when doing longer exercise

Perform low-to-moderate intensity levels of exercise through keto-adaptation Improving

health and losing more fat through regular exercise and low-carb eating Maintaining

blood glucose during exercise

Adapting the body to burning more fat, which might be able to help the body preserve glycogen in the muscles during exercise

Muscle Growth And Ketosis

We don't currently have research showing a specific benefit of ketogenic diets over higher carb diets for muscle growth during strength or high-intensity exercises. That being said, there are some studies show that in addition to using more fat as fuel, low- carb diets can also help preserve muscle glycogen for some athletes. Plus, a ketogenic diet has the advantage of teaching the body to more easily turn to fat burning for fuel.

However, that doesn't mean it's necessary to turn to a very high carb diet to see success in muscle growth and performance. In fact, a diet that is higher in protein and more moderate in carb intake might be the best for achieving ideal body composition and muscle growth for most active people and some sports athletes.

An Early Account Of Ketogenic Diet Performance

Let's take a second to travel back over a hundred years ago to one of the earliest recorded examples of a ketogenic diet for intense physical performance.

Benefits Of Ketosis For Athletes

A lower carb intake does have some potential benefits for certain types of athletes. For example:

Some research shows that the preservation of glycogen stores from a ketogenic diet can prevent endurance athletes from "hitting the wall" while performing endurance exercises.

Keto-adaptation can lead to less reliance on carbs during endurance exercise, which can help athletes during events where there is limited access to food or those who can't easily digest carbs during exercise.

A diet that promotes more fat loss is important for improve the ratio of fat to muscle, which is crucial for those looking to improve their exercise performance or meet certain weight goals for their sport, such as in wrestling, weightlifting, and boxing.

The practice of exercising while glycogen stores are low is a training technique popular for improving the function of mitochondria, enzymes, and fat usage to improve overall health and physical performance long-term.

Eating a ketogenic diet might also be a good diet practice for an athlete's off season as they maintain their health while resting.

While the jury is still out on the benefits of a ketogenic diet over a higher carb diet for all athletes, ketosis for physical performance can be helpful for those doing ultra- endurance or low-intensity exercise meant to maintain health.

WHAT IS KETO FLU

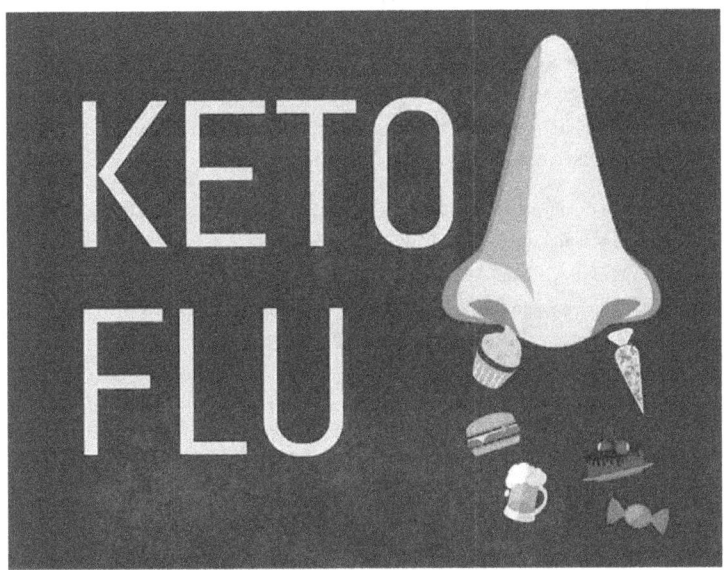

Many people have decided to try the ketogenic diet for weight loss. The most recent evidence shows that reducing your carbohydrate intake to a minimum may help you shed a few pounds, at least in the first few weeks to months. However, we don't really know whether, over the long term, achieving and maintaining ketosis is better for weight loss than other diets. Almost any intervention can cause undesirable consequences, and the ketogenic diet is no different. One of the most well-publicized complications of ketosis is something called "keto flu."

What is keto flu?

The so-called keto flu is a group of symptoms that may appear two to seven days after starting a ketogenic diet. Headache, foggy brain, fatigue, irritability, nausea, difficulty sleeping, and constipation are just some of the symptoms of this condition, which is not recognized by medicine. A search for this term yields not a single result on PubMed, the library of indexed medical research journals. On the other hand, an internet search will yield thousands of blogs and articles about keto flu.

It is tricky to describe exactly what happens after the diet change, because we are left with only our own observations and experiences. These symptoms may not even be unique to the ketogenic diet; some of my patients describe similar symptoms after they cut back on processed foods, or decide to follow an elimination or an anti-inflammatory diet.

What causes keto flu?

Well, we don't really know why some people feel so bad after this dietary change. Is it related to a detox factor? Is it due to a carb withdrawal? Is there an immunologic reaction? Or is this a result of a change in the gut microbiome? Whatever the reason is, it appears the symptoms attributed to the keto flu may happen, not to everyone but to some people, after "cleaning up" their diet.

What to do for keto flu?

If you decide for whatever reason to change your diet and feel tired and a little off, do not become exasperated and lose hope. Here are few tips:

Supercharge your cold and flu defenses!

Surprising secrets, smart strategies, and simple steps to keep your immune system at its cold-and-flu-fighting best

Get the tips to stay healthy

There is no need to go online and buy any expensive supplements. Many websites are trying to make big bucks selling products to make you feel better without any data to back up those claims.

Despite its name, this is not like the flu. You will not develop a fever and the symptoms can hardly ever make you incapacitated. If you feel very ill, consider visiting your doctor, as something else may be happening.

Make sure you drink plenty of water. Some diets can make you dehydrated.

Eat more often and make sure you have plenty of colorful vegetables. Switching from a standard American diet, rich in simple carbs, trans fats, and saturated fat, is a big change in how your cells use energy. Food is not only calories and energy, it is communication to your cells.

Do not give up if you are committed to a plan. You may feel exhausted for a few days, but at the end of a week, your energy level will most likely return to normal and you may feel even better.

If everything else fails, consider easing into the new diet more slowly, instead of "cold turkey."

Undesirable symptoms may show up in the first few days after changing what you eat. But this should not be the deciding factor when choosing what to put on your plate.

How To Get Rid Of The Keto Flu

The keto flu can make you feel miserable.

Luckily, there are ways to reduce its flu-like symptoms and help your body get through the transition period more easily.

Stay Hydrated

Drinking enough water is necessary for optimal health and can also help reduce symptoms.

A keto diet can cause you to rapidly shed water stores, increasing the risk of dehydration

This is because glycogen, the stored form of carbohydrates, binds to water in the body. When dietary carbohydrates are reduced, glycogen levels plummet and water is excreted from the body

Staying hydrated can help with symptoms like fatigue and muscle cramping

Replacing fluids is especially important when you are experiencing keto-flu-associated diarrhea, which can cause additional fluid loss

Avoid Strenuous Exercise

While exercise is important for staying healthy and keeping body weight in check, strenuous exercise should be avoided when experiencing keto-flu symptoms.

Fatigue, muscle cramps and stomach discomfort are common in the first week of following a ketogenic diet, so it may be a good idea to give your body a rest.

Activities like intense biking, running, weight lifting and strenuous workouts may have to be put on the back burner while your system adapts to new fuel sources.

While these types of exercise should be avoided if you are experiencing the keto flu, light activities like walking, yoga or leisurely biking may improve symptoms.

Replace Electrolytes

Replacing dietary electrolytes may help reduce keto-flu symptoms.

When following a ketogenic diet, levels of insulin, an important hormone that helps the body absorb glucose from the bloodstream, decrease.

When insulin levels decrease, the kidneys release excess sodium from the body

What's more, the keto diet restricts many foods that are high in potassium, including fruits, beans and starchy vegetables.

Getting adequate amounts of these important nutrients is an excellent way to power through the adaptation period of the diet.

Salting food to taste and including potassium-rich, keto-friendly foods like green leafy vegetables and avocados are an excellent way to ensure you are maintaining a healthy balance of electrolytes.

These foods are also high in magnesium, which may help reduce muscle cramps, sleep issues and headaches

Get Adequate Sleep

Fatigue and irritability are common complaints of people who are adapting to a ketogenic diet.

Lack of sleep causes levels of the stress hormone cortisol to rise in the body, which can negatively impact mood and make keto-flu symptoms worse

If you are having a difficult time falling or staying asleep, try one of the following tips:

Reduce caffeine intake: Caffeine is a stimulant that may negatively impact sleep. If you drink caffeinated beverages, only do so in the morning so your sleep is not affected

Cut out ambient light: Shut off cell phones, computers and televisions in the bedroom to create a dark environment and promote restful sleep

Take a bath: Adding Epsom salt or lavender essential oil to your bath is a relaxing way to wind down and get ready for sleep

Get up early: Waking at the same time every day and avoiding oversleeping may help normalize your sleep patterns and improve sleep quality over time

UNDERSTANDING NUTRIENT RATIOS

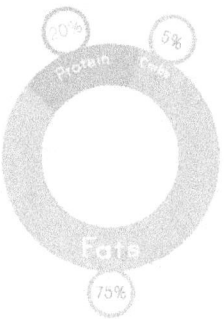

Keto macros are the most important aspect of the ketogenic diet. They include the three nutrients that your body needs in large amounts fat, protein, and carbs. Get them wrong and your chances of reaching ketosis are close to zero!

In this guide, we explain what macros are and how you can calculate your keto macros. We also offer practical bits of advice that can make meeting your keto macros a whole lot easier.

Calculating Keto Macros

The easiest way to calculate your keto macros is with a keto calculator. We've developed a precise keto calculator based on the standard ketogenic diet that will calculate you your keto macros in less than a minute. However, if you'd like to learn more about keto macros, including your daily allotment, keep reading.

What Are Macros?

Macros are nutrients that your body needs in large amounts in order to sustain wide range of metabolic processes. Medical and nutrition experts classify the following five nutrients as macros :

Carbohydrates

Proteins

Fats Fiber

Water

However, what most people refer to when talking about macros is carbohydrates, proteins, and fats. These three are also of great importance on a ketogenic diet. They are energy-providing nutrients whose total energy yield is defined in calories.

A balance in macros is also of huge importance for overall health. Studies show that eating too much or little of a single macro increases one's risk of obesity, heart disease, and diabetes. The worst offender of the three is carbs, but the one carrying the greatest stigma is fat (we'll talk more about that later).

Besides macronutrients, your body also needs micronutrients. Micronutrients are nutrients that you need to eat in smaller amounts, and they mostly include vitamins and minerals. It's easy to get adequate amounts of both micro and macronutrients from a well-planned ketogenic diet.

How to Calculate Macros For Keto

"Keto macros" is a term referring to the macronutrient ratio of a ketogenic diet. This ratio looks something like this:

60-75% of calories from fat

15-30% of calories from protein

5-10% of calories from carbs

This macronutrient ratio is different from what the medical community recommends and from what most people are used to. In fact, The Institute of Medicine recommends that active people get 45-65% of their energy from carbs, 10-35% from protein, and 20- 35% from fat.

So, what's the deal here? Well, the goal of a keto diet is different from that of standard health diets. On a keto diet, your goal is to radically change the way your body uses nutrients for energy production by placing the body into a metabolic state called ketosis. The standard diet, on the other hand, is meant to optimize the way your body already makes and uses food for energy.

There are many reasons why you'd want to induce ketosis, but the most sought-after is to force your body to burn fat, instead of glucose, for fuel. When your body does this, you lose excess body fat, become more energized, and experience greater mental clarity.

Below is a breakdown of each macro so you can better understand their function on the keto diet:

Carbohydrates

Carbohydrates are your body's preferred fuel source. The reason for this is that they are easy to break down and turn into energy. However, unlike proteins and fat, carbs are still not an essential nutrient.

Carbs are simply a cheap and convenient sources of energy. In the absence of carbs, your body is perfectly adapted to surviving on protein and fats. Not only that, but your body may just benefit from occasional carb restriction.

The biggest problem with carbs is that they're easy to overconsume. The typical Western diet is laden with all of the wrong carbs, and this is believed to be behind the global rise in metabolic diseases and obesity.

Another problem with carbs is that some can cause low-grade inflammation, a condition linked to things like cancer and cardiovascular diseases.

The keto diet minimizes carb intake to a level that will help your body burn fat and also maintain good health.

Protein

Protein is an essential macronutrient that the body needs to build and repair tissue. Proteins are large molecules consisting of amino acids. There are around 20 amino acids in nature, 9 of which are essential for human health. You can get essential amino acids from both plant and animal foods.

On a keto diet, you have to adjust your protein intake in accordance with your activity levels: the more active you are, the more protein you'll need. However, going overboard on protein can, and will, kick you out of ketosis because your body is able to turn a portion of the protein you eat into glucose.

On a positive note, one great thing about protein is that it keeps you feeling full for a long time because it takes longer to digest. Protein also boosts weight loss because your body actually burns calories to digest it. Finally, protein builds muscle tissue, which further increases your energy expenditure.

Fats

Fat is a central keto macro but also the reason behind much of today's nutrition controversy. Medical experts have been warning the public about the dangers of high-fat diets for decades. The fact of the matter is that fat is an essential nutrient that your body cannot do without. Eliminating it from your diet does more harm than good, and researchers have been saying this for at least two decades now after reevaluating the role of fat in health and disease.

What we now know about fat is that it:

Provides energy

Helps your body use fat-soluble vitamins (A, D, E, and K)

Maintains body temperature

Maintains healthy skin and hair Promotes

cell health

Accumulates toxins to protect internal organs

Supports hormone production

Fat is central to the ketogenic diet, helping the body make ketones to fuel your body and brain by replacing glucose. If you lower your calorie intake, your body will also start to use stored fat for energy.

Types of Fat

There are many different types of fat, some good and some bad.

Bad fats are trans fats found in excess in highly processed and fried food. Some margarines are also high in trans fats. Good fats are the monounsaturated and polyunsaturated fats found in plant oils. Saturated fats are also good, but some may not agree with this. Keto experts vouch for it as do many researchers and medical experts today.

Fats also contain essential and non-essential fatty acids. Essential fatty acids are alpha-linolenic acid (omega-3 fatty acids) and linoleic acid (omega-6 fatty acids). Your body can make other fatty acids from omega fats, but it cannot make omega fats on its own so you need to get them from food.

You can get essential fatty acids from a wide range of food sources. The best sources by far are fish, other seafood, nuts, plant oils, and seeds. Eating a variety of these foods is a foolproof way to meet your daily needs for omega fatty acids.

How to Calculate Macros for Keto

Keto macros are roughly the same for your most people. However, for maximum efficiency, you want keto macros to match your physique, needs, and goals. The easiest way to do that is by using a keto calculator.

However, there are other ways to calculate and keep track of your keto macros:

1. Start with net carbs

Net carbs are total carbs minus fiber. Calculating them is important on a keto diet because your body makes glucose only from net carbs. Fiber has no effect on your blood glucose levels whatsoever, so feel free to load up on it.

Take a look at nutrition labels on food packaging or online for fresh produce.

Your daily intake of net carbs should not exceed 30 grams. This is the upper limit you can reach before being kicked out of ketosis. However, eating around 20 grams a day is optimal for most people. Athletes may need to eat more to have enough energy during workouts.

2. Move on to proteins

Your protein allowance on a keto diet will depend on whether you want to build muscle, lose weight, and your body fat percentage*. As a rule of thumb, you need around 1.5 to 2.5 grams of protein per kilogram of muscle mass to maintain or gain muscle**. That's 0.7 to 1 grams of protein per pound of muscle mass. You will need less if you are not trying to gain muscle. Below is a formula to help you determine your daily protein allowance.

a) Start by calculating your body fat by using the following formula (the example provided is for someone weighing 160 pounds with a 20 % body fat percentage):

160 pounds x 0.20 (20 %) = 32 pounds of body fat

b) Subtract your body fat percentage from 100 to get your lean muscle mass percentage: 100 - 20 percent (of body fat) = 80% of muscle mass

c) Then divide this by 100 to get the decimal for your muscle weight: 80 /

100 = 0.80

d) Finally, multiply this decimal by total weight to calculate your total lean mass weight: 160 (pounds) x 0.80 = 128 of lean mass

e) To calculate your daily protein allowance, simply multiply your muscle mass by gram of protein. The formula goes like this:

128 pounds (of muscle mass) x 0.7-1 grams (protein per pound of muscle mass) = 89- 128 grams of protein

3. Finish with fats

After you've determined your daily carb and protein allowance, you'll have to calculate how much fat you should eat. This will depend on whether you want to lose or maintain weight. To maintain weight, you need to eat more fat than to lose weight.

The easiest way to calculate your daily fat allowance is, of course, by using a keto calculator. The calculator will provide you with your daily allowance of fat in grams. If you want to know how many calories you are taking in, consider the following facts:

Protein and carbohydrates contain 4 calories per gram Fat

contains 9 calories per gram.

This means that if, say, a keto (macros) calculator shows you need to eat 200 grams of fat that 1,800 of your daily calories should come from fat:

200 grams (of fat) x 9 calories (per gram) = 1,800 calories from fat

On average, women need to eat around 2,000 and men around 2,500 calories per day. But these numbers vary greatly depending on your age, weight, and physical activity levels along with your goals (if you're trying to lose weight or gain muscle mass).

A surplus of 500 calories will either help you maintain muscle mass or total weight, while a deficiency will help you lose body fat. However, we need to mention that many keto experts doubt the necessity of counting calories on a keto diet. The reason being that fat is highly satiating, so going overboard is difficult. Another reason is that the ketogenic diet in itself suppresses appetite [8] but also has a strong thermic effect.

How to Calculate Food Macros

You know that some foods are high in fat and low in carbs, while others are the exact opposite (think avocado vs. white rice). But that doesn't really help you on a practical level. You want to know how many keto macros you're taking in with your meals.

Calculating keto macros in food items as well as whole meals is pretty easy. However, we need to warn you that it can be time-consuming when you first start doing this. Nevertheless, calculating macros is an important step in getting your ratio just right. You can do this by using nutrition facts from reliable websites.

Take for example Myfitnesspal.com. The website offers nutrition facts for a wide range of food items. Simply enter a food item in the search bar and the website will give you precise nutrition facts per serving, including total fat, total carbs, dietary fiber, protein, and calories.

Besides Myfitnesspal.com, you can use our food list of keto-approved foods and visit our Foods & Nutrition Blogs to learn more about keto foods. Once you have a list of keto foods ready, use nutrition facts websites to calculate your keto macros.

Example:

1 medium avocado (250 calories)

Fat: 23 grams

Net carbs: 5 grams (15 grams total carbs - 10 grams fiber),

Protein: 0 grams

Served with one poached egg (74 calories)

Fat: 5 grams

Net carbs: 0 grams

Protein: 6 grams

Topped with a teaspoon of olive oil (40 calories)

Fat: 5 grams

Net carbs: 0 grams

Protein: 0 grams

From this 364-calorie meal, you get a total of 33 grams of fat, 5 grams of net carbs, and 6 grams of protein. Make similar lists for all your meals and keep them close when you plan your meals.

Tips & Tricks for Meeting Macros

Stick to whole foods

Highly processed foods contain hidden ingredients that can sabotage your dieting efforts. In other words, you never know what you are taking in when munching on packaged foods labeled "low-carb" or "keto". The keto diet is all about clean eating as this supports good health, and most importantly – helps you stay within your keto macros.

Plan your meals

Planning meals is non-negotiable on a keto diet. You simply can't make food choices on spur of the moment because then you won't be able to track your keto macros. Planning meals is time-consuming at first. But once you have your list ready, most of your planning is already done.

Find a ready-made meal plan

An even easier way to meet your keto macros is to use existing meal plans. Many keto websites offer weekly, monthly, and even half-year meal plans. This takes away much of the hassle that you initial go through when trying to plan meals and meet keto macros. Make sure you only use meal plans from reputable sources with good ratings.

Take-Home Message

Keto macros are the essence of a ketogenic diet. You want to balance them out perfectly to reach your goals and feel good along the way. This can be a bit tricky as it involves plenty of planning and mathematics.

But once you have your macros set and your meal plan in place, keto dieting will become your second nature. Use our keto calculator, read our informative blog posts, and consider our guidance and tips given here when trying to meet your macros.

DANGERS OF EATING KETO

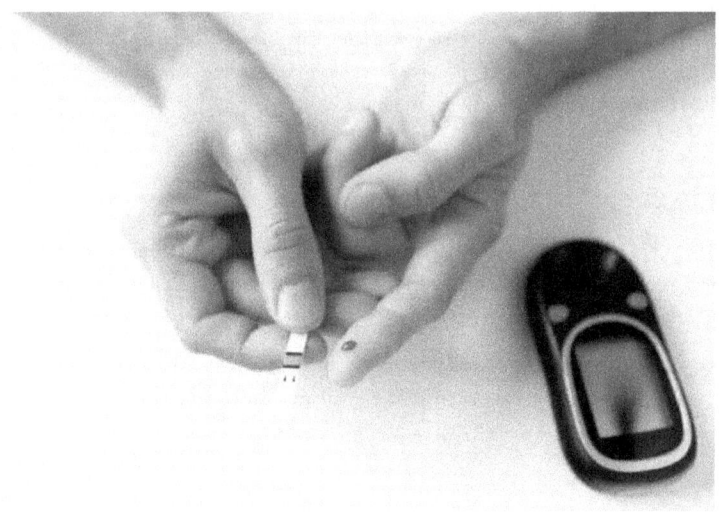

Here are some potential challenges and dangers of eating keto.

1.   Athletic Performance Impediments: For those people who train heavy and hard, going keto might cramp your style. As important as protein is for muscle growth, carbs also play an equally critical role by releasing insulin to drive that protein into muscles faster. It also helps us build up glycogen stores for longer training sessions, runs or hikes. One comprehensive review of the literature in sports nutrition found that while research is lacking on the long-term impacts of the keto diet, in the short term, the keto diet is inferior to other diet protocols on anaerobic, aerobic and in some cases even strength performance measures.

2.   Keto "Flu": Your body isn't accustomed to using ketones on the regular, so when you make the switch, you tend to feel unwell. The keto diet also influences electrolyte balance, resulting in brain fog, headaches, nausea and fatigue. Keto dieters also consistently complain about getting bad-smelling breath, sweat and pee as a result of the by-product of fat metabolism (acetone) seeping out. Thankfully, this effect is just temporary, so just know you won't have to spend your life smelling rank.

3.   Constipation: No one likes to feel backed up, and sadly if you're not careful about your diet choices when going keto, it could become a regular concern. One 10-year (albeit small) study looking at the effects of a keto diet on young children found that 65 percent experienced digestive woes. Thankfully, going keto is not a life sentence for problem bowels. Since you're cutting out whole grains and fruit (two of the most common sources of fiber), aim to up your fiber-rich veggies, and consider a supplement.

4.   Nutrition Deficiencies: As with any super-restrictive regimen, when you cut food out, there's a good chance you'll be missing something big. Here's what you need to keep an eye open for.

5.   Sodium: Believe it or not, depending on your diet, you may be low on salt. When carb intake is low and insulin isn't being excreted, the kidneys absorb less sodium and potassium and excrete more as waste, leaving you feeling dizzy, fatigued and grumpy. Rather than reaching for more processed food, try seasoning your food a little more liberally with sea salt.

6.   Potassium: With the approved list of foods being so brief, you might not be getting in enough fruits and veggies on keto. One of the biggest impacts? A potassium deficiency— and all of the lovely constipation and muscle cramps that accompanies it. Aim to up

your intake of foods like spinach, avocado, tomatoes, kale and mushrooms to get your potassium fix.

7.   Vitamin C: Most of our vitamin C intake comes from a nice array of fruits, so if you're cutting all of that out, you'll have to make sure you're keeping your veggies up to compensate. Reach for more broccoli, Brussels sprouts, cauliflower and cabbage to ensure you get your fill.

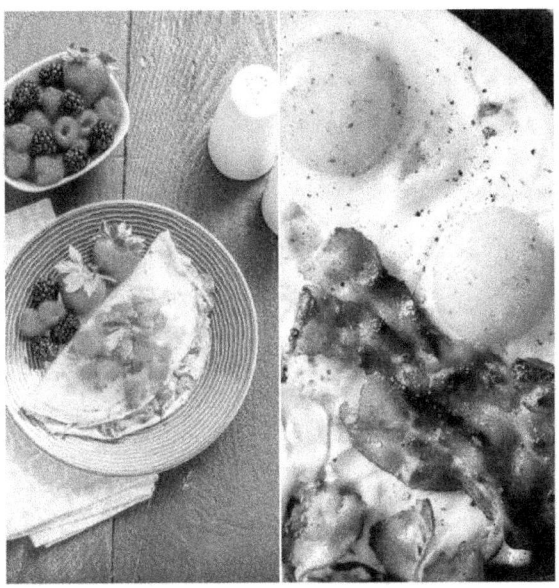

Obesity rivals smoking as the number one cause of preventable death. One reason is the dramatic rise in the diabetes risk often accompanying weight gain. So, are you interested in starting up a new diet plan, one aimed to not only help you lose weight but to control your blood sugar better? Chances are you are searching for the best options available. Two you may come across as they are trendy in today's times are the ketogenic diet and the paleo diet. Many people actually get confused between these as they do tend to be similar so it can be hard to differentiate between them.

Let us compare so you can see which one is right for you...

Carb Sources. First, let's talk carb sources as this is where the two diets vastly differ...

with the paleo diet plan, your carb sources are going to be any fresh fruit, along with sweet potatoes. Together, you can quickly achieve 100 grams or more of carbohydrates between these two foods.

the keto diet, on the other hand, your only carb source is leafy greens, and even those are restricted.

So one of the most significant differences between the ketogenic diet and the paleo diet plan is the ketogenic diet is deficient in carbohydrates while the paleo is not. You can make the paleo diet very low carb if you want, but it is not by default. There is more flexibility in food choices.

Calorie Counting. Next, we come to calorie counting. This is also a place where the two diets differ considerably.

With the keto diet, you will be calorie and macro counting quite heavily. You need to hit specific targets...

30% total protein intake, 5%

carbohydrate intake and 65%

dietary fat intake.

If you do not reach these targets, you are not going to move into the "state of ketosis," which is the entire point of this diet plan.

With the paleo diet, there are no strict rules around this. While you can count calories if you want, you do not have to. Obviously, your fat loss results will likely be better if you do monitor calories to some degree since calories do dictate whether you gain or lose body fat, but it is not essential.

Exercise Fuel Availability. Which brings us to our next point - exercise fuel availability. To be able to exercise with intensity, you need carbohydrates in your diet plan. You cannot get fuel availability if you are not eating carbohydrate-rich foods - that means the keto diet is not going to support intense exercise sessions. For this reason, the keto diet will not be optimal for most people. Exercise is an integral part of staying healthy, so it is strongly recommended you exercise and do not follow a diet that limits exercise.

Of course, you can do the targeted ketogenic diet or the cyclic ketogenic diet, both of which have you including carbohydrates in the diet at some point...

the targeted ketogenic diet has you eating carbohydrates just before starting your workout session while

the cyclic ketogenic diet calls for you to eat a larger dose of carbs over the weekend, which are designed to sustain you through the rest of the week.

If you follow either of these, you can choose any carbohydrates you wish; it does not necessarily have to be just sweet potatoes or fruit.

There you have some critical differences between this two approaches...

the ketogenic diet is one focusing more on tracking macros and is intended to assist with fat loss while

the paleo diet focuses more on good food choices and health and hopes weight loss comes as a result.

Although managing Type 2 diabetes can be very challenging, it is not a condition you must just live with. Make simple changes to your daily routine - include exercise to help lower both your blood sugar levels and your weight.

Does A Keto Diet Help Lower Blood Sugar Levels

Is a ketogenic diet safe for people who have received a diagnosis of Type 2 diabetes? The food recommended for people with high blood sugar encourages weight loss: a ketogenic diet has high amounts of fat and is low in carbs, so it is mystifying how such a high-fat diet is an option for alleviating high blood sugar.

The ketogenic diet underlines a low intake of carbohydrates and increased consumption of fat and protein. The body then breaks down fat by a process called "ketosis," and produces a source of fuel called ketones. Usually, the diet improves blood sugar levels while decreasing the body's need for insulin. The diet initially was developed for epilepsy treatment, but the kinds of food and the eating pattern it highlights, are being studied for the benefit of those with Type 2 diabetes.

The ketogenic diet contains foods such as... pasta,

fruits, and bread

as a source of body energy. People with Type 2 diabetes suffer from high and unstable blood sugar levels, and the keto diet helps them by allowing the body to preserve their blood sugar at a low healthy level.

How does a keto diet help many with Type 2 diabetes? In 2016, the Journal of Obesity and Eating Disorders published a review suggesting a keto diet may help people with diabetes by improving their A1c test results, more than a calorie diet.

The ketogenic diet places emphasis on the consumption of more protein and fat, making you feel less hungry and therefore leading to weight loss. Protein and fat take longer to digest than carbohydrates and helps to keep energy levels up.

In a nutshell, the ketogenic diet... lowers

blood sugar,

enhances insulin sensitivity and

promotes less dependency on medications.

The Keto Diet Plan. Ketogenic diets are stringent, but if adhered to correctly they can provide a nourishing and healthful nutrition routine. It is about staying away from carbohydrate foods likely to spike blood sugar levels.

People with Type 2 diabetes are often advised to focus on this diet plan as it consists of a mix of low carbohydrate foods, high-fat content, and moderate protein. It is also important because it avoids high-processed foods and indulges in lightly processed and healthy foods.

A ketogenic diet should consist of these types of food...

low-carb vegetables: eat vegetables with every meal. Avoid starchy vegetables like corn and potatoes.

eggs: they contain a low amount of carbohydrates and are a high source of protein.

meats: eat fatty meats but avoid excessive amounts. High amounts of protein plus low carbohydrates can lead to the liver converting protein into glucose, thus causing the person to come out of ketosis.

fish: an excellent source of protein.

Eat from healthy sources of fat like avocados, seeds, nuts, and olive oil.

Although managing your disease can be very challenging, Type 2 diabetes is not a condition you must just live with. You can make simple changes to your daily routine and lower both your weight and your blood sugar levels. Hang in there, the longer you do it, the easier it gets.

Should You Use A Ketogenic Diet Plan

As someone who is working hard to control or prevent Type 2 diabetes, one diet you may have heard about is the ketogenic or keto diet plan. This diet is a very low carbohydrate diet plan consisting of around...

5% total carbohydrates, 30%

protein, and a whopping 65%

dietary fat.

If there is one thing this diet will do, its help to control your blood sugar levels. This said, there is more to eating well than just controlling your blood sugar.

Let's go over some of the main reasons why this diet doesn't always stack up to be as great as it sounds...

1. You'll Be Lacking Dietary Fiber. The first big problem with the ketogenic diet is you'll be seriously lacking in dietary fiber. Almost all vegetables are cut from this plan (apart from the very low-carb varieties), and fruits are definitely not permitted. High fiber grains are also out of the equation, so this leaves you with primarily protein and fats - two foods containing no fiber at all.

2. You'll Be Low In Energy. Another big issue with the ketogenic diet is you'll be low in energy to carry out your exercise program. Your body can only utilize glucose as a fuel source for very intense exercise and if you aren't taking in carbohydrates, you'll have no glucose available.

3. You May Suffer Brain Fog. Those who are using the ketogenic diet may also find they suffer from brain fog. Again, this is thanks to the fact your brain primarily runs off glucose.

4. Your Antioxidant Status Will Decline. Finally, the last issue with the ketogenic diet is due to the lack of fruit and vegetable content - your antioxidant status is going to sharply decline.

So keep these points in mind as the diet comes with some risks. The ketogenic diet converts fat instead of sugar into energy. It was first created as a treatment for epilepsy but now the effects of the diet are being looked at to help Type 2 diabetics lower their blood sugar. Make sure you discuss the diet with your doctor before making any dietary chan

RELATIONSHIP BETWEEN DIABETES AND KETOACIDOSIS

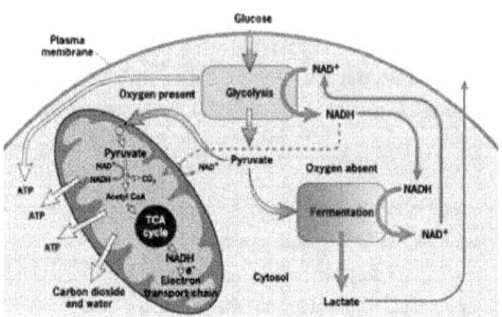

For those with type 1 diabetes, ketoacidosis is a common, severe complication. Diabetic ketoacidosis occurs when the blood is very acidic and the blood glucose levels are very high.

The prefix "keto" refers to the substance known in the body as "ketones." Ketones are created by your body during the process of breaking down of fat. When the levels of ketones in the blood stream get really high the blood becomes very acidic.

In many cases, it is the acid blood that first indicates to doctors that a patient may have type 1 diabetes. If the doctors already know you have type 1 diabetes, they are not so surprised when you show symptoms of diabetic ketoacidosis in your tests. However, on average those with type 1 diabetes do not get diagnosed with ketoacidosis until they are at least 40 years old.

Ketoacidosis Is More Common in Type 1 Diabetics Than Type 2 Diabetics

People who have type 2 diabetes have reduced amounts of insulin production into their bloodstreams. People who have type 1 diabetes have dramatically reduced to know insulin production into their bloodstreams. This accounts for why those with type 1 diabetes are far more likely to develop ketoacidosis than those with type 2 diabetes.

Signs & Symptoms of Diabetic Ketoacidosis

1. Rapid Breathing

Your body may actually become acidic enough that it tries to use the lungs as a location to excrete acid. During this rapid breathing process, often referred to as "Kassmaul Breathing," your lungs are literally filled with acid from the bloodstream in a desperate attempt by your body to balance out the blood.

2. Nauseous Vomiting

As acids build up in your body it is very common to feel nauseous and to eventually begin vomiting. This may be another desperate attempt by your body to get rid of some acid. However, your bodily fluids may become very unbalanced, leading to further complications.

3. Chronic Drowsiness

The thick, acidic blood that gathers in the brain can cause you to become very drowsy and sluggish.

4. Weak Muscles

As ketoacidosis sets in your bloodstream will do an even worse job of distributing and using glucose where it is needed. As a result your muscles will not have the fuel they need to function the way they normally would. Every movement may seem like a chor

THE TRUTH ABOUT CARBS

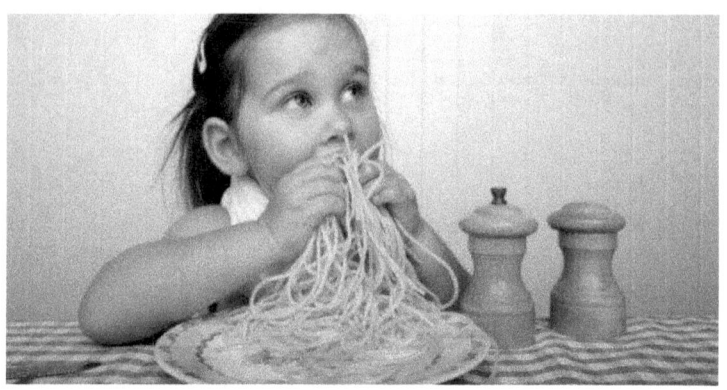

Carbohydrates are one of 3 macronutrients (nutrients that form a large part of our diet) found in food – the others being fat and protein.

Hardly any foods contain only 1 nutrient, and most are a combination of carbohydrates, fats and proteins in varying amounts.

There are 3 different types of carbohydrates found in food: sugar, starch and fibre.

Sugar

The type of sugars most adults and children in the UK eat too much of are called free sugars.

These are the sugars added to food or drinks, including sugars in biscuits, chocolate, flavoured yoghurts, breakfast cereals and fizzy drinks.

Sugars in honey, syrups (such as maple, agave and golden), nectars (such as blossom), and unsweetened fruit juices, vegetable juices and smoothies occur naturally, but still count as free sugars.

Sugar found naturally in milk, fruit and vegetables does not count.

Starch

Starch is found in foods that come from plants. Starchy foods, such as bread, rice, potatoes and pasta, provide a slow and steady release of energy throughout the day.

Fibre

Fibre is the name given to the diverse range of compounds found in the cell walls of foods that come from plants.

Good sources of fibre include vegetables with skins on, wholegrain bread, wholewheat pasta, and pulses (beans and lentils).

Why do we need carbs?

Carbohydrates are important to your health for a number of reasons.

Energy

Carbohydrates should be the body's main source of energy in a healthy, balanced diet, providing about 4kcal (17kJ) per gram.

They're broken down into glucose (sugar) before being absorbed into the bloodstream. From there, the glucose enters the body's cells with the help of insulin.

Glucose is used by your body for energy, fuelling all of your activities, whether going for a run or simply breathing.

Unused glucose can be converted to glycogen found in the liver and muscles.

If more glucose is consumed than can be stored as glycogen, it's converted to fat for long-term storage of energy.

Higher fibre starchy carbohydrates release sugar into the blood more slowly than sugary foods and drinks.

Disease risk

Fruit and vegetables, pulses, wholegrain and wholewheat varieties of starchy foods, and potatoes eaten with their skins on, are good sources of fibre.

Fibre is an important part of a healthy, balanced diet. It can promote good bowel health, reduce the risk of constipation, and some forms of fibre have been shown to reduce cholesterol levels.

Research shows diets high in fibre are associated with a lower risk of cardiovascular disease, type 2 diabetes and bowel cancer.

Many people don't get enough fibre. On average, most adults in the UK get about 19g of fibre a day. We're advised to eat an average of 30g a day.

Calorie intake

Carbohydrate contains fewer calories gram for gram than fat and starchy foods can be a good source of fibre, which means they can be a useful part of maintaining a healthy weight.

By replacing fatty, sugary foods and drinks with higher fibre starchy foods, it's more likely you'll reduce the number of calories in your diet.

Also, high-fibre foods add bulk to your meal, helping you feel full. "You still need to watch your portion sizes to avoid overeating," says Sian.

"Also watch the amount of fat you add when cooking and serving them: this increases the calorie content."

Should I cut out carbohydrates?

While we can most certainly survive without sugar, it would be quite difficult to eliminate carbohydrates entirely from your diet.

Carbohydrates are the body's main source of energy. In their absence, your body will use protein and fat for energy.

It may also be hard to get enough fibre, which is important for long-term health.

Healthy sources of carbohydrates, such as higher fibre starchy foods, vegetables, fruits and legumes, are also an important source of nutrients, such as calcium, iron and B vitamins.

Significantly reducing carbohydrates from your diet in the long term could put you at increased risk of insufficient intakes of certain nutrients, potentially leading to health problems.

Cutting out carbohydrates from your diet could put you at increased risk of a deficiency in certain nutrients, leading to health problems, unless you're able to make up for the nutritional shortfall with healthy substitutes.

Replacing carbohydrates with fats and higher fat sources of protein could increase your intake of saturated fat, which can raise the amount of cholesterol in your blood a risk factor for heart disease.

When you're low on glucose, the body breaks down stored fat to convert it into energy. This process causes a build-up of ketones in the blood, resulting in ketosis.

Ketosis as a result of a low-carbohydrate diet can be linked, at least in the short term, to headaches, weakness, nausea, dehydration, dizziness and irritability.

Try to limit the amount of sugary foods you eat and instead include healthier sources of carbohydrate in your diet, such as wholegrains, potatoes, vegetables, fruits, legumes and lower fat dairy products.

Don't protein and fat provide energy?

While carbohydrates, fat and protein are all sources of energy in the diet, the amount of energy each one provides varies:

carbohydrate provides: about 4kcal (17kJ) per gram protein

provides: 4kcal (17kJ) per gram

fat provides: 9kcal (37kJ) per gram

In the absence of carbohydrates in the diet, your body will convert protein (or other non-carbohydrate substances) into glucose, so it's not just carbohydrates that can raise your blood sugar and insulin levels.

If you consume more calories than you burn from whatever source, you'll gain weight.

So cutting out carbohydrates or fat doesn't necessarily mean cutting out calories if you're replacing them with other foods containing the same number of calories.

Are carbohydrates more filling than protein?

Carbohydrates and protein contain roughly the same number of calories per gram.

But other factors influence the sensation of feeling full, such as the type, variety and amount of food eaten, as well as eating behavior and environmental factors, like serving sizes and the availability of food choices.

118

The sensation of feeling full can also vary from person to person. Among other things, protein-rich foods can help you feel full, and we should have some beans, pulses, fish, eggs, meat and other protein foods as part of a healthy, balanced diet.

But we shouldn't eat too much of these foods. Remember that starchy foods should make up about a third of the food we eat and we all need to eat more fruit and vegetables.

How much carbohydrate should I eat?

The government's healthy eating advice, illustrated by the Eatwell Guide, recommends that just over a third of your diet should be made up of starchy foods, such as potatoes, bread, rice and pasta, and over another third should be fruit and vegetables.

This means that over half of your daily calorie intake should come from starchy foods, fruit and vegetables.

What carbohydrates should I be eating?

These are usually high in sugar and calories, which can increase the risk of tooth decay and contribute to weight gain if you eat them too often, while providing few other nutrients.

Fruit, vegetables, pulses and starchy foods (especially higher fibre varieties) provide a wider range of nutrients (such as vitamins and minerals), which are beneficial to health.

The fibre in these foods can help keep your bowels healthy and adds bulk to your meal, helping you feel full.

How can I increase my fibre intake?

To increase the amount of fibre in your diet, aim for at least 5 portions of a variety of fruit and veg a day.

Go for higher fibre varieties of starchy foods and eat potatoes with skins on. Try to aim for an average intake of 30g of fibre a day.

Here are some examples of the typical fibre content in some common foods: 2

breakfast wheat biscuits (approx. 37.5g) – 3.6g of fibre

1 slice of wholemeal bread – 2.5g (1 slice of white bread – 0.9g) 80g of

cooked wholewheat pasta – 4.2g

1 medium (180g) baked potato (with skin) – 4.7g

80g (4 heaped tablespoons) of cooked runner beans – 1.6g 80g

(3 heaped tablespoons) of cooked carrots – 2.2g

1 small cob (3 heaped tablespoons) of sweetcorn – 2.2g 200g

of baked beans – 9.8g

1 medium orange – 1.9g 1

medium banana – 1.4g

Can eating low glycaemic index (GI) foods help me lose weight?

The glycaemic index (GI) is a rating system for foods containing carbohydrates. It shows how quickly each food affects glucose (sugar) levels in your blood when that food is eaten on its own.

Some low-GI foods, such as wholegrain foods, fruit, vegetables, beans and lentils, are foods we should eat as part of a healthy, balanced diet.

But using GI to decide whether foods, or a combination of foods, are healthy or can help with weight reduction can be misleading.

Although low-GI foods cause blood sugar levels to rise and fall slowly, which may help you to feel fuller for longer, not all low-GI foods are healthy.

For example, watermelon and parsnips are high-GI foods, while chocolate cake has a lower GI value.

And the way a food is cooked and what you eat it with as part of a meal will change the GI rating.

This means GI alone isn't a reliable way of deciding whether foods, or combinations of foods, are healthy or will help you lose weight.

Do carbohydrates make you fat?

Any food can cause weight gain if you overeat. Whether your diet is high in fat or high in carbohydrates, if you frequently consume more energy than your body uses you're likely to put on weight.

In fact, gram for gram, carbohydrate contains fewer than half the calories of fat. Wholegrain varieties of starchy foods are good sources of fibre. Foods high in fibre add bulk to your meal and help you feel full.

But foods high in sugar are often high in calories, and eating these foods too often can contribute to you becoming overweight.

There's some evidence that diets high in sugar are associated with an increased energy content of the diet overall, which over time can lead to weight gain.

Can cutting out wheat help me lose weight?

Some people point to bread and other wheat-based foods as the main culprit for their weight gain.

Wheat is found in a wide range of foods, from bread, pasta and pizza to cereals and many other foods.

But there's not enough evidence that foods that contain wheat are any more likely to cause weight gain than any other food.

Unless you have a diagnosed health condition, such as wheat allergy, wheat sensitivity or coeliac disease, there's little evidence that cutting out wheat and other grains from your diet would benefit your health.

Grains, especially wholegrains, are an important part of a healthy, balanced diet.

Wholegrain, wholemeal and brown breads give us energy and contain B vitamins, vitamin E, fibre and a wide range of minerals.

White bread also contains a range of vitamins and minerals, but it has less fibre than wholegrain, wholemeal or brown breads.

If you prefer white bread, look for higher fibre options. Grains are also naturally low in fat.

Find out if cutting out bread could help ease bloating or other digestive symptoms

Should people with diabetes avoid carbs?

People with diabetes should try to eat a healthy, balanced diet, as shown in the Eatwell Guide.

They should also include higher fibre starchy foods at every meal. Steer clear of cutting out entire food groups.

It's recommended that everyone with diabetes sees a registered dietitian for specific advice on their food choices. Your GP can refer you to a registered dietitian.

There's some evidence that suggests low-carbohydrate diets can lead to weight loss and improvements in blood glucose control in people with type 2 diabetes in the short term.

But it's not clear whether the diet is a safe and effective way to manage type 2 diabetes in the long term.

Weight loss from a low-carbohydrate diet may be because of a reduced intake of calories overall and not specifically as a result of eating less carbohydrate.

There also isn't enough evidence to support the use of low-carbohydrate diets in people with type 1 diabetes.

What's the role of carbohydrates in exercise?

Carbohydrates, fat and protein all provide energy, but exercising muscles rely on carbohydrates as their main source of fuel.

But muscles have limited carbohydrate stores (glycogen) and need to be topped up regularly to keep your energy up.

A diet low in carbohydrates can lead to a lack of energy during exercise, early fatigue and delayed recovery.

●

When is the best time to eat carbohydrates?

There's little scientific evidence that one time is better than any other.

It's recommended that you base all your meals around starchy carbohydrate foods and you try to choose higher fibre wholegrain varieties when you can.

30 DAYS KETOGENIC DIET PLAN

WEEK1

In my eyes, simplicity is key for someone that is just starting out on a low carb diet. You don't want it to be a difficult transition (kitchen-wise), because it will be hard to just get rid of your cravings.

The first signs of ketosis are known as the "keto flu" where headaches, brain fogginess, fatigue, and the like can really rile your body up. Make sure that you're drinking plenty of waterand eating plenty of salt. The ketogenic diet is a natural diuretic and you'll be peeing more than normal. Take into account that you're peeing out electrolytes, and you can guess that you'll be having a thumping headache in no time. Keeping your salt intake and water intake high enough is very important, allowing your body to re-hydrate and re-supply your electrolytes. Doing this will help with the headaches, if not get rid of them completely.

If you need to, drink water with a sprinkling of salt in it. Just keep drinking water (I recommend 4 liters a day), and keep eating salt. It will help, trust me. If you're worried about high blood pressure and salt, don't be! Recent studies show that the sodium intake and blood pressure are not as correlated as we so once believed.

Breakfast.

For breakfast, you want to do something that's quick, easy, tasty, and of course – gives you leftovers. I suggest starting day 1 on a weekend. This way, you can make something that will last you for the entire week. The first week is all about simplicity. Nobody wants to be making breakfast before work, and we're not going to be doing that either!

Lunch.

We're also going to keep it simple here. Most of the time, it'll be salad and meat, slathered in high fat dressings and calling it a day. We don't want to get too rowdy here. You can use leftover meat from previous nights or use easy accessible canned chicken/fish. If you do use canned meats, try to read the labels and get the one that uses the least (or no) additives!

Dinner.

Dinner will be a combination of leafy greens (normally broccoli and spinach) with some meat. Again, we'll be going high on the fat and moderate on the protein.

P.S. No dessert for the first 2 weeks.

Week 2

Wow, week 1 is over. I hope you're still doing well on the diet and have found it pretty easy breezy to keep on track with everything!

This week we're going to be keeping it simple for breakfast again. We're going to introduce ketoproof coffee. It's a mixture of coconut oil, butter, and heavy cream in your coffee. If this repulses you – and I know some of you are saying "WHAT?" – just put some trust in me!

This concoction is not as strange as it sounds. Butter, after all, is made out of cream. So when you blend the oil, butter, and cream together it just adds a decadent richness to your coffee that I am quite sure you'll really like!

Breakfast.

For breakfast, we are going to change it up a bit. Here's where we introduce ketoproof coffee. Now, don't get me wrong – I know some of you won't like it. If you're not a fan of coffee, then try it with tea. If you're not a fan of the taste (which is very rare), then try making a mixture of the ingredients by themselves and eating it like that. So, why ketoproof coffee?

Fat Loss. Plain and simple, the consumption of medium-chain triglycerides (MCT) has been shown to lead to greater losses in adipose tissue (fat tissue), in both animals and humans.

Fats! Do I even need to explain this one? Eating fat has been shown to lead to greater amounts of energy, more efficient energy usage, and more effective weight loss. Not to mention, it's the main component of this diet.

More Energy. Studies have shown that the rapid rate of oxidation in MCFAs (Medium Chain Fatty Acids) leads to an increase in energy expenditure. Primarily, MCFAs are converted into ketones (our best friends), are absorbed differently in the body compared to regular oils, and give us more overall energy.

Feel free to add sweetener and spices to this if you're not the biggest fan of the taste. Cinnamon, stevia, vanilla extract. Whatever you'd like to make it great tasting. You can even switch up the taste each and every day so you don't get bored!

If this is your first time drinking ketoproof coffee, I suggest taking 1-2 hours or so to drink it down. Normally when people have a large exposure to coconut oil and they're not used to it, it can make them go to the bathroom quite often. Make sure you build a tolerance to coconut oil before drinking it within a 20 minute time frame.

Lunch.

We're still keeping simple here. We can incorporate more meat from the previous night of cooking into each lunch we do. Green vegetables and high fat dressings (or vinaigrettes) are key. Making sure to balance out the fats with the amounts of protein is very important.

Dinner.

Dinner, again, will be pretty simplistic. Meats, vegetables, high fat dressings are the center of our life. Maybe even a slathering of butter on our vegetables since we're getting friskier. Don't over think things in the first 2 weeks; simple is success.

P.S. No dessert for this week either, but we'll be delving into that next week!

Week 3

This week we're introducing a slight fast. We're going to get full on fats in the morning and fast all the way until dinner time. Not only are there a myriad of health benefits to this, it's also easier on our eating schedule (and cooking schedule). I suggest eating (rather, drinking) your breakfast at 7am and then eating dinner at 7pm. Keeping 12 hours between your 2 meals. This will help put your body into a fasted state.

In a fasting state, our bodies can break down extra fat that's stored for the energy it needs. When we're in ketosis, our body already mimics a fasting state, being that we have little to no glucose in our bloodstream, so we use the fats in our bodies as energy.

Intermittent fasting is using the same reasoning – instead of using the fats we are eating to gain energy, we are using our stored fat. That being said, you might think it's great – you can just fast and lose more weight. You have to take into account that later on, you will need to eat extra fat in order to keep out of a starvation mode state.

There are a number of benefits shown that come from intermittent fasting. Some of these include blood lipid levels, longevity, and the much needed mental clarity.

If you find that you can't do a fast, then no big deal. Go back to week 1 and experiment as you see fit. You can eat what you want as long as it fits into your macros.

This is where things start to get more fun – less to worry about, more deliciousness to cook!

Breakfast.

We're going full on fats with breakfast, just like we did last week. This time we'll double the amount of ketoproof coffee (or tea) we drink, meaning we double the amount of coconut oil, butter, and heavy cream. It should come to quite a lot of calories, and should definitely keep us full all the way to dinner. Remember to continue drinking water like a fiend to make sure you're staying hydrated.

Lunch.

No lunch, oh no! Don't worry – the fats from the morning should keep you feeling energized and full all the way through lunch. Normally people start hitting a wall at first at around 2pm, so make sure you have plenty of water to drink, drink, and drink.

Dinner.

Well, dinner is staying the same. Meats, vegetables, and fats are almost always going to be the dinnertime norm. But don't worry – we'll mix in some bread-y type things!

And guess what, we get to eat dessert this week! Woo! We'll be creating some low carb and great tasting treats that will reward you ever so much for doing the fasting. Sweets, treats, and losing weight lucky us, right?

Week 4

This week we're getting stricter with our fasting. We had a full week of intermittent fasting and now we're going to skip breakfast and lunch. Water is our BEST friend here! Don't forget that you can drink coffee, tea, flavored water, and the like to get your liquids in. Keep drinking to make sure you're not thinking about your stomach. It MIGHT start growling, just ignore it – your body will adjust with time.

Now, if you're the kind of person that can't fast then you can go back and follow week 2 again. That's no big deal. Though fasting does take some time for the body to get used to, so I suggest putting your best efforts into it. Not only are the health benefits fantastic, the self-control that you gain from doing so is really a great thing.

This is by far my favorite week because it most closely resembles how I eat on a daily basis. I normally set a window of 6 hours for myself to eat in. From waking up until 5pm, I fast. After that, I am open to eating until 11pm. This is where the real fun begins. Eating copious amounts of food and being full all the way through the next day.

You get to start experimenting more with dessert and dinner. You get to snack as you please inside your window and best of all – you get to eat that protein laden chicken that you've been missing so much of!

Breakfast.

We're fasting! Black coffee if you're a caffeine addict like me. Tea, if you are not into the coffee so much. Tea can add great health benefits like coffee also. Some of the great benefits of green tea are:

Polyphenols – These function as antioxidants in your body. The most powerful antioxidant in green tea is Epigallocatechin gallate (EGCG), which has shown to be effective against fatigue.

Improved Brain Function – Not only does green tea contain caffeine, it also contains L-theanine, which is an amino acid. L-theanine increases your GABA activity, which improves anxiety, dopamine, and alpha waves.

Increased Metabolic Rate – Green tea has been shown to improve your metabolic rate. In combination with the caffeine, this can lead up to 15% increased fat oxidization.

Lunch.

Water, water, and then some more water. You don't get to eat lunch and you don't get to eat breakfast. So make sure you keep yourself VERY hydrated. It's imperative here that you do a good job with your hydration. Remember – I recommend 4 liters a day.

Dinner.

Lots and lots of food with dessert to cover the bases! Dinner is a fantastic time for me. I suggest breaking your fast with a small snack, then after 30-45 minutes eat to your hearts content. Normally I need 2 meals to get to my macros, and I think you'll need to do the same.

Week 5

This is where we have to depart! Sorry to say but you're on your own. You should have plenty of leftovers that are frozen, ready, and waiting! I know a lot of you out there have trouble with timing and are busy people so making sure that some nights you make extras to freeze is important. All those leftovers you have in the freezer? Use them up. Create your own meal plan, at first using this as a guide, and then completely doing it yourself. Once you get the hang of it, it'll be a sinch – I promise you!!

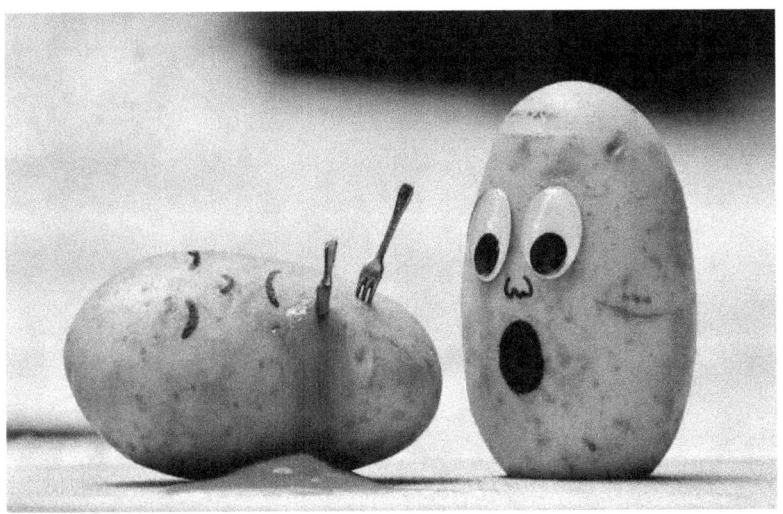

Eating a high amount of fat, moderate protein, and low amount of carbs can have a massive impact on your health lowering your cholesterol, body weight, blood sugar, and raising your energy and mood levels.

A ketogenic diet can be hard to fathom in the beginning but isn't as hard as it's made out to be. The transition can be a little bit tough, but the growing popularity of the clean eating movement makes it easier and easier to find available low-carb foods.

Keep it straightforward and strict. You usually see better results in people who restrict their carb intake further. Try to keep your carbs as low as possible for the first month of keto. Keep it strict by cutting out excess sweets and artificial sweeteners altogether (like diet soda). Cutting these out dramatically decreases sugar cravings.

Drink water and supplement electrolytes. Most common problems come from dehydration or lack of electrolytes. When you start keto (and even in the long run), make sure that you drink plenty of water, salt your foods, and take a multivitamin. If you're still experiencing issues, you can order electrolyte supplements individually.

Track what you eat. It's so easy to over-consume on carbs when they're hidden in just about everything you pick up. Keeping track of what you eat helps control your carb intake and keep yourself accountable.

Anti-Inflammatory Diet For Beginners

Table of Contents

INTRODUCTION

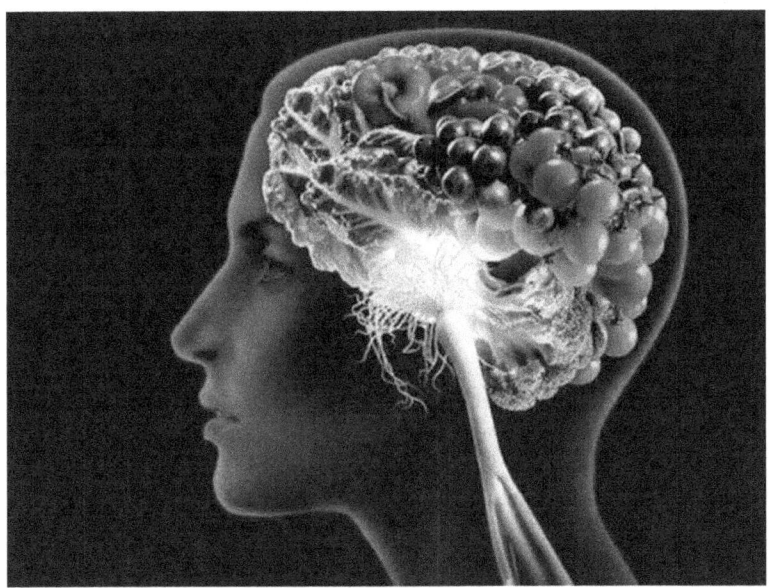

One of the most incredible and complex parts of the human body is the immune system. The immune system is able to recognize foreign substances like viruses and bacteria that might do our body harm.

It's important to know that there are two main parts of the immune system. The first is innate immunity and you are born with it totally intact; its job is to protect you against outside threats through its protective barriers like mucus and stomach acid. Fevers and the cough reflex are some other example of antigens that the innate immunity handles.

The second type of immunity makes up the adaptive immune system and it's constantly developing as you develop in life. Each time you are exposed to a germ or illness, your adaptive immune system keeps a record of it and helps your body build up a pre-programmed defense. And then, ideally, it won't make you sick the next time you come into contact with it. This adaptive immune process involves a complex system of chemicals, cells, and biological pathways that make up one of the great wonders of the human body.

The immune system and inflammation go hand in hand, and causing an inflammatory response is one major way the immune system responds to a threat and starts to fight off bacteria or tissue damage.

WHAT IS INFLAMMATION

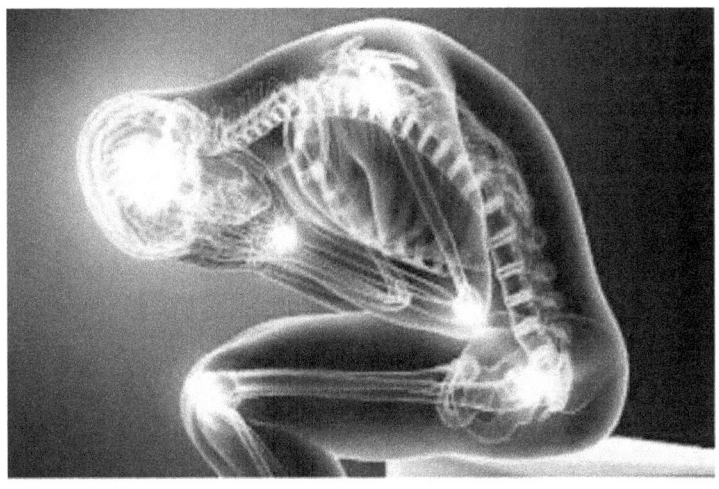

Inflammation is a natural process with the biological purpose to initiate healing by increasing circulation. It is a complex process involving both the immune system and vascular system and the interplay of various chemical mediators. Increased circulation brings white blood cells and nourishment to the site of injury or infection so that invading pathogens are killed and damage may be repaired. Characteristic signs of inflammation include pain (dolor), heat (calor), swelling (tumor) and redness (rubor).

When Inflammation Goes Awry:

While some inflammation is beneficial and appropriate for healing, chronic or excessive inflammation, serving no purpose produces damage. Chronic inflammation has a bad reputation because it is implicated in various disease processes including (but not limited to)...

- autoimmune diseases

- arthritis

- diabetes

- Alzheimer's disease

- atherosclerosis (hardening of arteries that leads to heart attack and stroke)

- ADD and ADHD

- allergies & asthma

- cancers

- inflammatory bowel disease

Soft tissue swelling and chemical mediators involved in inflammation can also irritate nerve endings, contributing to pain.

What is the Anti-Inflammatory Diet?

It is a well-known fact that different foods are metabolized differently, some promoting inflammation and others reducing it. The purpose of the anti-inflammatory diet is to promote optimal health and healing by choosing foods that reduce inflammation. If one can successfully control excessive inflammation through natural means (like through diet), it reduces one's dependence on anti-inflammatory medications that have unwanted and unhealthy side effects and don't solve the underlying problem. While anti-inflammatory medications (such as NSAIDs) is a quick fix to ease symptoms, they ultimately weaken the immune system by damaging the gastrointestinal tract which plays an important role in immune system function.

Anti-inflammatory Diet Basics:

In general, eat an abundance of fresh vegetables and fruits, whole grains, anti-inflammatory fats and nuts while limiting processed foods, meat protein, milk products, refined sugars, artificial colors/flavors/sweeteners and food sensitivities.

Vegetables:

Enjoy an abundance of fresh vegetables and fruits in a variety of colors (preferably organic). Fruits and vegetables are full of vitamins, minerals, antioxidants and fiber which give the body the essential building blocks for health. Examples include beans, squash, lintels, sweet potatoes, cruciferous vegetables, avocados, dark leafy greens... There are so many choices! As for fruits, pineapple and papaya are particularly good because they are high in bromelain, a powerful natural anti-inflammatory. Fruits and vegetables also make great, healthy snacks.

Avoid / Limit:

Avoid produce that is not grown organically. Toxic chemical residues from herbicides and pesticides can remain and when ingested are foreign irritants to the system. Many crops in North America are also genetically engineered and are put on the market without rigorous scientific study to determine safety for human consumption. Independent research is finally being done to show toxic effects of consuming genetically modified organisms. Foreign DNA is randomly inserted into the genome of a crop. Examples include herbicide resistant corn and soy which are resistant to the herbicide Roundup, made by Monsanto. Roughly 90% of all corn and soy sold in North America is genetically modified. Also be aware of derivatives of genetically modified ingredients (such as corn starch and corn syrup etc.). It has also been suggested that consuming GMOs is a contributing factor to the rise in allergies as our bodies are recognizing these food substances as foreign. By choosing items with the "certified organic" label, you avoid both GMOs and toxic herbicides/pesticides.

For some people, vegetables in the nightshade family may pose a concern. Examples of nightshade vegetables include tomatoes, peppers, potatoes and eggplant. Nightshades contain alkaloids which are thought to exacerbate inflammation and joint damage in certain susceptible individuals with arthritis (though research is conflicting). Thus, for some individuals, limiting or avoiding nightshade vegetables may be beneficial.

Fats:

Enjoy healthy, anti-inflammatory fats including olive oil, coconut oil, avocados, nuts, salmon and sardines. In humans, there are two essential fatty acids, alpha-linolenic acid (an omega-3) and linoleic acid (an omega-6). These are "essential" because they are required for good health but the body does not synthesize them. Omega-3 fats are anti-inflammatory. Omega-6 fats can be pro-inflammatory or anti-inflammatory (as it can be metabolized by two different pathways). Researchers suggest that keeping the ratio of omega-6 to omega-3 between 2:1 and 4:1 is best for health. The modern diet tends to be high in omega-6 as it is abundantly available in cooking oils. Thus, including rich sources of omega-3 is important (such as fish, flax and walnuts especially).

Avoid / Limit:

Fats to limit or avoid include margarine, butter, shortening, hydrogenated oils, trans fats, saturated fats, and milk fat. Omega-6 fats are very high in corn oil, safflower oil and sunflower oil. Trans fats are linked with inflammatory diseases.

Meat:

In general, limit animal proteins because they tend to acidify the body and also promote inflammation. When selecting animal protein, enjoy fish, poultry (especially free-range and organically raised), lamb and omega-3 eggs.

Avoid / Limit:

Limit beef, pork, shellfish and factory farmed eggs. In general, grass-fed is superior to grain-fed. Avoid charred foods, smoked foods and cold cuts. Cold cuts contain nitrates and nitrites which promote cancer. Barbequed foods contain polycyclic aromatic hydrocarbons (PAHs) and heterocyclic amines (HCAs) which also promote cancer.

Dairy:

Enjoy dairy substitutes in moderation (such as almond milk).

Avoid / Limit:

Avoid or limit dairy products in general. This includes milk, yogurt, cheese and ice cream. As we age, we lose the enzyme that digests dairy, resulting in lactose intolerance and inflammation. The milk protein, casein, is also acidifying which (despite what many people are brought up thinking) robs the bones of calcium.

Grains:

Enjoy whole grains as opposed to refined grains. Refined grains are grains in which the germ and bran have been removed. This means there is loss of fiber, minerals and vitamins. In other words, the good stuff is removed in exchange for a longer shelf life. Some good examples of healthy grains include (organic) whole wheat/oats/bulgar/coucous, quinoa and whole oats (like steel-cut oats).

Whole grains are also a rich source of complex carbohydrates. Complex carbohydrates (as opposed to simple sugars) will prevent spikes in your blood sugar level. Sugar promotes inflammation.

Avoid / Limit:

Avoid or limit refined carbohydrates such as white bread, pastries, sweet things and pastas.

Nuts:

Enjoy nuts and nut butters such as almonds, walnuts, sesame seeds, pumpkin seeds and flax.

Avoid / Limit:

Avoid any specific nut allergies.

Beverages:

Enjoy plenty of pure, filtered water (avoiding chlorine, fluoride and other contaminants which are irritants that promote inflammation). Other great choices are lemon water and herbal teas.

Avoid / Limit:

Avoid sugary sodas, fruit juice (with sugar added) and milk.

Spices:

Many spices reduce inflammation. Some great examples are turmeric, oregano, rosemary, ginger, garlic and cinnamon. Bioflavenoids and polyphenols reduce inflammation and fight free radicals. Cayenne pepper is also anti-inflammatory, as it contains capsicum. Capsicum is often used in pain-relief creams.

Sweeteners:

Enjoy stevia, molasses, maple syrup or honey as better alternatives for refined sugar.

Avoid / Limit:

Avoid refined sugar, fructose and especially high fructose corn syrup which promote inflammation. Avoid artificial sweeteners.

Other:

Enjoy fermented foods such as kimchi, miso soup and sauerkraut. Fermented foods are probiotic and help to rebuild the immune system by supporting healthy microflora in the gut and to reduce inflammation. Fermented foods also tend to be easy to digest and are also factories for B vitamins.

Avoid / Limit:

In general, eliminate processed foods, artificial colors, artificial flavors and preservatives. Also avoid foods that you have a known sensitivity or allergy to as this promotes inflammation. Low grade sensitivities are easy to miss, so if you're unsure, have a food allergy test. Some of the most common problem foods include wheat (gluten), corn, soy, milk and nuts.

Everything we need for health, can be found in nature. We just need to choose well. If you need help and ideas of what to eat, there are plenty of anti-inflammatory diet recipe books available.

What Else Can You Do to Reduce Inflammation?

- Chiropractic care boosts immune system and reduces inflammation!

- Reduce exposure to environmental toxins (such as smoke)

- Reduce stress (5)

- Certain types of exercise reduce inflammation - specifically, long term, gradually progressive training, avoiding over-exertion (6)

ABOUT THE ANTI-INFLAMMATORY DIET

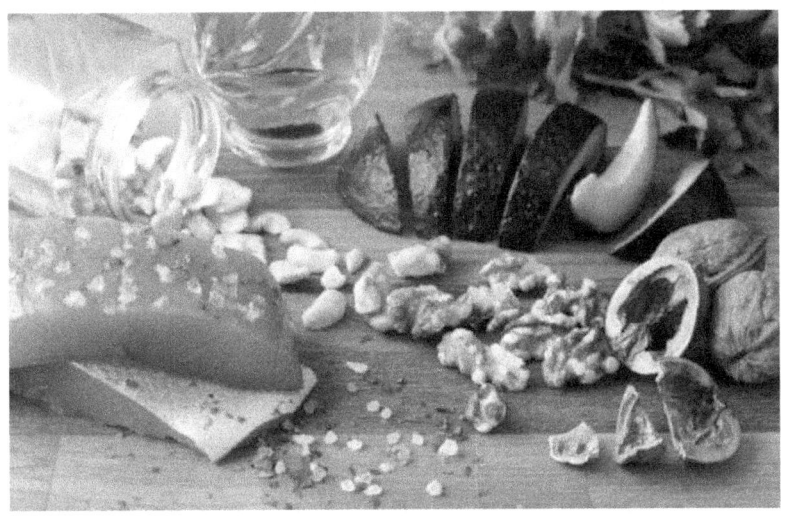

Anti-inflammatory foods are getting tons of hype these days. In fact, just about everyone is using the term "inflammation," from your cardiologist to Tom and Gisele! But keep your baloney detector on.

11   Inflammatory diets are also a thing.

The saturated fat added sugar and sodium in refined carbs and processed snacks make your body's cells work overtime to get their regular job done. Doctors can identify inflammation using biomarkers of oxidative stress, the result of biological processes that cause organ tissue damage. Diet, exercise and smoking status can affect inflammation, but so do uncontrollable causes like autoimmune diseases.

12   It's not just for weight loss.

Anti-inflammatory eating is more of a disease prevention plan. A overwhelming amount of research has shown that people who eat anti-inflammatory foods are at significantly lower risk of developing chronic disease. They're also more likely to maintain healthy weights.

13   Anti-inflammatory foods are everywhere.

The anti-inflammatory diet is often considered a Mediterranean diet, since they recommend the similar foods: Veggies, fruit, whole grains, nuts, seeds, oils, legumes, low-fat dairy and fish. The flavonoids in plants are specifically linked to protecting your body's cells from damage. Both produces and lean protein sources like beans and seafood also contain good-for-you polyunsaturated and monounsaturated fats.

14   You may have these hidden signs of inflammation.

You can't feel inflammation but, if you know what symptoms to look for, you can catch it early, before health conditions emerge. Potential inflammatory warning signs include digestive issues, intermittent joint pain, new food sensitivities, belly fat, worsening allergies, brain fog, unexplained fatigue, moodiness, sleep problems, and rashes.

15   It's inclusive, not exclusive.

Traditional diets always talk about what you can't eat, but when it comes to anti-inflammatory diets, more is more. Colorful foods like leafy greens (spinach, kale), cruciferous veggies (broccoli, cauliflower), carotenoids (tomatoes, carrots) and anthocyanins (beets, berries) are all anti-inflammatory staples.

16 You won't feel hungry.

The plant-based powerhouses known as pulses are an excellent way to incorporate antioxidant- and mineral-rich foods into your everyday life. Dry peas, beans, chickpeas and lentils combine lean protein, unsaturated fats and fiber, filling you up without messing with your diet.

17 Wine and coffee are encouraged.

When it comes to decreasing your risk of Alzheimer's, cardiovascular disease and diabetes, light to moderate alcohol intake of any kind can help. Packed with flavonoids and antioxidants, coffee beans not only ward off cognitive decline, but also boost brain function and stimulation of the central nervous system. Just steer clear of sweetened drinks sugary beverages can increase inflammation!

18 Your mood could get a boost.

Women of childbearing age eat 50% less fish than they should, largely due to previous confusion about prenatal effects. The truth is 12 ounces a week can provide a whole host of anti-inflammatory benefits. Plus, the omega-3's in fish have been linked to a lower risk of depression and reduced anxiety symptoms. Some of our favorite picks include tuna, salmon, sardines, anchovies and other white fish.

19 It's filled with flavor.

Turmeric offers powerful anti inflammatory benefits, says Dr. Corey Kirschner, of the Whole Body Cure, an anti-inflammatory diet plan from our partners at Prevention. Supercharge its anti inflammatory effects by combining it with black pepper, which helps to increase the amount of curcumin (the active ingredient in turmeric) your body can absorb. Turmeric is also fat soluble, he says, so you'll increase your absorption by combining it with a healthy fat like olive oil.

20 Cooking oils are a-okay.

Extra-virgin olive oil is filled with polyphenols, antioxidant-compounds linked to maintaining cell integrity and improving blood flow throughout your body. Canola oil, made from rapeseed, is another anti-inflammatory staple.

21 Conscious indulgences are key.

Ultimately, the anti-inflammatory diet emphasizes real foods as close to nature as possible. But since indulgence is a key part of any eating plan, try treating yourself to about 200 calories of chocolate per day. Research says that eating chocolate regularly may also help maintain a normal BMI. Plus, it can help you cut back on other processed treats.

22 You can try a whole body approach.

Prevention's Whole Body Cure includes 60+ anti-inflammatory recipes, along with the detailed advice you need to reverse chronic inflammation — no prescription required.

23 tomato salad

Just one meal or snack or heck, even a weekend full of fried food cannot induce a state of "inflammation." However, an anti-inflammatory diet may help many people lose weight because it's chock-full of nutrient-dense and delicious foods.

An Anti-Inflammatory Diet For Leaky Gut Disease

Leaky gut disease or leaky gut syndrome is a condition that can be caused by antibiotics, infections, parasites, toxins, or poor diet. The significant feature of the condition is alteration or damage to the bowel lining. As the lining becomes more permeable than normal it allows microbes, undigested food, waste, toxins, or large macromolecules to enter. Some researchers believe that these substances have a direct affect on the body; others think the problem is an immune reaction to those substances.

Whatever has caused it for you, you probably just wish the symptoms -- everything from acne and indigestion to anxiety and fatigue to joint pain and constipation, to name a few - would go away. Unfortunately, that wish can lead to treating just the symptoms. If you have Leaky Gut Disease, however, it's important that you don't just address the symptoms. You need to focus on the root causes of the condition.

One -- if not the main one -- of these root causes is diet. While practitioners disagree on a lot of things about Leaky Gut Disease (whether it even really exists, for example), the diet primarily recommended for those suffering from it - the anti-inflammatory diet - is generally acknowledged to be a healthy one for almost everyone.

The anti-inflammatory diet isn't really a diet; it's more of an eating plan. And if you do a little research, you'll find that there's not just one anti-inflammatory diet; there are several, each with a different spin. For our purposes here, I've tried to present what is a "generic" version. This version does share with the others the concept that continued and out-of-control inflammation leads to illness and that following an eating plan that avoids inflaming the body promotes health and can help prevent disease.

In general an anti-inflammatory diet includes:

Plenty of fruits and vegetables

Plenty of whole grains (e.g., brown rice, bulgur wheat)

Lean protein (e.g., chicken, fish)

Anti-inflammatory spices (e.g., curry, ginger)

Omega-3 fatty acids (such as those found in fish, fish oil supplements, and walnuts)

A reduction in

Refined carbohydrates (e,g., pasta, white rice)

Red meat and full-fat dairy foods

Saturated and trans fats

No refined or processed foods

Many who endorse this diet also urge that you avoid refined sugar and products that contain it as well as caffeine and alcohol. And while drugs don't really fall into the diet category, have your doctor review your prescriptions and monitor your own use of OTC drugs, especially NSAIDS.

One word of caution regarding this plan: The effects you experience (i.e., an improvement in your symptoms) will not be as immediate as they would be if you treated yourself with medications. You probably need to give the anti-inflammatory diet at least two weeks versus the hour or two a medicine might take. On the other side, this diet might have a bonus effect not usually found in medications: weight loss!

HISTORY AND PHYSICAL

Age: Increasing age is positively correlated with elevated levels of several inflammatory molecules. The age-associated increase in inflammatory molecules may be due to mitochondrial dysfunction or free radical accumulation over time and other age-related factors like increase in visceral body fat.

Obesity: Many studies reported that fat tissue is an endocrine organ, secreting multiple adipokines and other inflammatory mediators. Some reports show that body mass index of an individual is proportional to the amount of pro-inflammatory cytokines secreted. Metabolic syndrome typifies this well.

Diet: Diet rich in saturated fat, trans-fats, or refined sugar is associated with higher production of pro-inflammatory molecules, especially in individuals with diabetes or overweight individuals.

Smoking: Cigarette smoking is associated with lowering the production of anti-inflammatory molecules and inducing inflammation.

Low Sex Hormones: Studies show that sex hormones like testosterone and estrogen can suppress the production and secretion of several pro-inflammatory markers and it has been observed that maintaining sex hormone levels reduces the risk of several inflammatory diseases.

Stress and Sleep Disorders: Both physical and emotional stress is associated with inflammatory cytokine release. Stress can also cause sleep disorders. Since individuals with irregular sleep schedules are more likely to have chronic inflammation than consistent sleepers, the sleep disorder is also considered as one of the independent risk factors for chronic inflammation.

What is chronic Inflammation?

To back up for a moment, let me give you a very brief primer on inflammation. It's a complex system in our bodies with an ever-growing list of identified components, but the big picture is that it occurs in two main ways. It can be a self-limited response to an injury or infection, for example if you get a paper-cut or a sprained ankle. You'll notice redness, pain, warmth and swelling in the area. But once all the cells from the inflammatory response have done their job and the injury is healed, that inflammation disappears. That's the kind of inflammation you want to happen.

The other kind of inflammation, called chronic inflammation, is the problematic one. It may occur if the immune system is trying to fend off an infection, like Lyme disease, but isn't having success. Or it may occur if the immune system becomes confused, such as in someone who has antibodies to gluten that also end up attacking other parts of the body that resemble gluten. Inflammation also happens when the immune system senses that something isn't right, such as when LDL cholesterol makes its way into the lining of an artery. White blood cells follow, but instead of fixing the problem, they inadvertently make it worse by making the plaque unstable and more likely to rupture

Symptoms of Chronic Inflammation

Some of the common signs and symptoms that develop during chronic inflammation are listed below.

Body pain

Constant fatigue and insomnia

Depression, anxiety and mood disorders

Gastrointestinal complications like constipation, diarrhea, and acid reflux

Weight gain

Frequent infections

Evaluation

Tests for Chronic Inflammation

Unfortunately, there are no highly effective laboratory measures to assess patients for chronic inflammation and diagnoses are only undertaken when the inflammation occurs in association with another medical condition.

The best test to confirm clinically chronic inflammation is serum protein electrophoresis (SPE) which shows concomitant hypoalbuminemia and polyclonal increase in all gamma globulins (polyclonal gammopathy).

The two blood tests that are inexpensive and good markers of systemic inflammation include high-sensitivity C-reactive protein (hsCRP) and fibrinogen. High levels of hs-

CRP indicate inflammation, but it is not a specific marker for chronic inflammation since it is also elevated in acute inflammation resulting from a recent injury or sickness. The normal serum levels for hsCRP is less than 0.55 mg/L in men and less than 1.0 mg/L in women. The normal levels of fibrinogen are 200 to 300 mg/dl. SAA (Serum Amyloid A) can also mark inflammation but is not a standardized test.

Detecting pro-inflammatory cytokines like tumor necrosis factor-alpha (TNF-alpha), interleukin-1 beta (IL-1beta), interleukin-6 (IL-6), and interleukin-8 (IL-8) is an expensive method but may identify specific factors causing chronic inflammation. Again, the assays are not standardized like hs-CRP, fibrinogen, and SPE.

Treatment / Management

Many dietary and lifestyle changes may be helpful in removing inflammation triggers and reducing chronic inflammation as listed below. The most effective is weight loss.

Low-glycemic diet: Diet with a high glycemic index is related to high risk of stroke, coronary heart disease, and type 2 diabetes mellitus. It is beneficial to limit consumption of inflammation-promoting foods like sodas, refined carbohydrates, fructose corn syrup in a diet.

Reduce intake of total, saturated fat and trans fats: Some dietary saturated and synthetic trans-fats aggravate inflammation, while omega-3 polyunsaturated fats appear to be anti-inflammatory. Processed and packaged foods that contain trans fats such as processed seed and vegetable oils, baked goods (like soybean and corn oil) should be reduced from the diet.

Fruits and vegetables: Blueberries, apples, Brussels sprouts, cabbage, broccoli, and cauliflower, that are high in natural antioxidants and polyphenols and other anti-inflammatory compounds, may protect against inflammation.

Fiber: High intake of dietary soluble and insoluble fiber is associated with lowering levels of IL-6 and TNF-alpha.

Nuts: such as almonds is associated with lowering risk of cardiovascular disease and diabetes.

Green and black tea polyphenols: Tea polyphenols are associated with a reduction in CRP in human clinical studies.

Curcumin: a constituent of turmeric causes significant patient improvements in several inflammatory diseases especially in animal models.

Fish Oil: The richest source of the omega-3 fatty acids. Higher intake of omega-3 fatty acids is associated with lowering levels of TNF-alpha, CRP, and IL-6.

Mung bean: Rich in flavonoids (particularly vitexin and isovitexin). It is traditional food and herbal medicine known for its anti-inflammatory effects.

Micronutrients: Magnesium, vitamin D, vitamin E, zinc and selenium). Magnesium is listed as one of the most anti-inflammatory dietary factors, and its intake is associated with lowering of hsCRP, IL-6, and TNF-alpha activity. Vitamin D exerts its anti-inflammatory activity by suppressing inflammatory mediators such as prostaglandins and nuclear factor kappa-light-chain-enhancer of activated B cells. Vitamin E, zinc, and selenium act as antioxidants in the body.

Sesame Lignans: Sesame oil consumption reduces the synthesis of prostaglandin, leukotrienes, and thromboxanes and is known for its potential hypotensive activity.

Physical Exercise

In human clinical trials, it is shown that energy expenditure through exercise lowers multiple pro-inflammatory molecules and cytokines independently of weight loss.

Conventional Drugs to Combat Chronic Inflammation

Metformin is commonly used in the treatment of type II diabetic patients with dyslipidemia and low-grade inflammation. The anti-inflammatory activity of Metformin is evident by reductions in circulating TNF-alpha, IL-1beta, CRP, and fibrinogen in these patients.

Non-steroidal anti-inflammatory drugs (NSAIDs) like naproxen, ibuprofen, and aspirin acts by inhibiting an enzyme cyclooxygenase (COX) that contributes to inflammation and are mostly used to alleviate the pain caused by inflammation in patients with arthritis.

Statins are anti-inflammatory as they reduce multiple circulating and cellular biomediators of inflammation. This pleiotropic effect appears to contribute in part to the reduction in cardiovascular events.

Corticosteroids also prevent several mechanisms involved in inflammation. Glucocorticoids are prescribed for inflammatory conditions including inflammatory arthritis, systemic lupus, sarcoidosis, and asthma.

Herbal supplements like ginger, turmeric, cannabis, hyssop, and Harpagophytum procumbens are shown to have anti-inflammatory properties however one should always consult with a doctor before their use and caution should be taken for using some herbs like hyssop and cannabis.

Differential Diagnosis

It is important to realize that chronic inflammation is not a specific disease but a mechanistic process. The diseases associated with chronic inflammation are multiple and include CVD, diabetes, malignancy, auto-immune disease, chronic hepatic and renal disease, etc. Hence a good history, physical examination, and routine laboratory tests (glucose, creatinine, liver function, rheumatoid factor, complete blood count, antinuclear antibodies) can confirm or rule out most of the differential diagnoses. Also, pertinent imaging studies will be helpful in certain circumstances, e.g., Inflammatory bowel disease or serum protein electrophoresis for polyclonal gammopathy.

Complications

Although chronic inflammation progresses silently, it is the cause of most chronic diseases and presents a major threat to the health and longevity of individuals. Inflammation is considered a major contributor to several diseases.

Cardiovascular diseases: Many clinical studies have shown strong and consistent relationships between markers of inflammation such as hsCRP and cardiovascular disease prediction. Furthermore, Atherosclerosis is a pro-inflammatory state with all the features of chronic low-grade inflammation and leads to increase cardiovascular events such as myocardial infarction, stroke, among others.

Cancer: Chronic low-level inflammation also appears to participate in many types of cancer such as kidney, prostate, ovarian, hepatocellular, pancreatic, colorectal, lung, and mesothelioma.

Diabetes: Immune cells like macrophages infiltrate pancreatic tissues releasing pro-inflammatory molecules in diabetic individuals. Both are circulating and cellular biomarkers underscore that diabetes is a chronic inflammatory disease. Chronic complications linked with diabetes include both microvascular and macrovascular complications. Diabetes not only increases the risk of macrovascular complications like strokes and heart attacks but also the microvascular complications like diabetic retinopathy, neuropathy, and nephropathy.

Rheumatoid arthritis: It is thought to be initiated by an infectious agent or an environmental factor like exposure to cigarette smoke which induces a local inflammatory response in joints, infiltration of immune cells and release of cytokines.

Allergic asthma: A complex, chronic inflammatory disorder associated with inappropriate immune response and inflammation in conducting airways involving a decline in airway function and tissue remodeling.

Chronic obstructive pulmonary disease (COPD): An obstructive lung disease, develops as a chronic inflammatory response to inspired irritants and characterized by long-term breathing problems.

Alzheimer: In older adults, chronic low-level inflammation is linked to cognitive decline and dementia.

Chronic kidney disease (CKD): Low-grade inflammation is a common feature of chronic kidney disease. It can lead to the retention of several pro-inflammatory molecules in the blood and contributes to the progression of CKD and mortality.

Inflammatory Bowel Disease (IBD) is a group of chronic inflammatory disorders of the digestive tract. It can develop as ulcerative colitis causing long-lasting inflammation and ulcers in the lining of large intestine and rectum or Crohn's disease characterized by inflammation of the lining of digestive tract dispersing into affected tissues such as mouth, esophagus, stomach and the anus.

Deterrence and Patient Education

Chronic inflammation can have a deleterious effect on the body and is a key factor causing almost all chronic degenerative diseases. The following are some of the most effective ways to prevent chronic inflammation.

Increase uptake of anti-inflammatory foods: It is important to avoid eating simple sugars, refined carbohydrates, high-glycemic foods, trans fats, and hydrogenated oils. Consuming whole grains, natural foods, plenty of vegetables and fruits such as avocados, cherries, kale, and fatty fish like salmon is helpful in defeating inflammation.

Minimize intake of antibiotics and NSAIDs: Use of antibiotics, antacids, and NSAIDs should be avoided as it could harm the microbiome in the gut causing inflammation in intestinal walls known as leaky gut which in turn releases toxins and triggers chronic, body-wide inflammation.

Exercise regularly to maintain an optimum weight: It is largely known that adipose tissue in obese or overweight individuals induces low-grade systemic inflammation. Regular exercise is helpful not only in controlling weight but also decreasing the risk of cardiovascular diseases and strengthening the heart, muscles, and bones.

Sleep longer: Overnight sleep (ideally at least 7 to 8 hours) helps stimulating human growth hormones and testosterone in the body to rebuild itself.

Stress Less: Chronic psychological stress is linked to greater risk for depression, heart disease and body losing its ability to regulate the inflammatory response and normal defense. Yoga and meditation are helpful in alleviating stress-induced inflammation and its harmful effects on the body.

Features

Most of the features of acute inflammation continue as the inflammation becomes chronic, including expansion of blood vessels (vasodilation), increase in blood flow, capillary permeability and migration of neutrophils into the infected tissue through the capillary wall (diapedesis). However, the composition of the white blood cells changes soon and the macrophages and lymphocytes begin to replace short-lived neutrophils. Thus the hallmarks of chronic inflammation are the infiltration of the primary inflammatory cells such as macrophages, lymphocytes, and plasma cells in the tissue site, producing inflammatory cytokines, growth factors, enzymes and hence contributing to the progression of tissue damage and secondary repair including fibrosis and granuloma formation, etc.

Types of Chronic Inflammation

Nonspecific proliferative: Characterized by the presence of non-specific granulation tissue formed by infiltration of mononuclear cells (lymphocytes, macrophages, plasma cells) and proliferation of fibroblasts, connective tissue, vessels and epithelial cells, for example, an inflammatory polyp-like nasal or cervical polyp and lung abscess.

Granulomatous inflammation: A specific type of chronic inflammation characterized by the presence of distinct nodular lesions or granulomas formed with an aggregation of activated macrophages or its derived cell called epithelioid cells usually surrounded by lymphocytes. The macrophages or epithelioid cells inside the granulomas often coalesce to form Langhans or giant cells such as foreign body, Aschoff, Reed-Sternberg and Tumor giant cells. There are two types:

Granuloma formed due to a foreign body or T-cell mediated immune response is termed as foreign body granuloma, for example, silicosis

Granuloma that are formed from chronic infection is termed as infectious granuloma, for example, tuberculosis and leprosy.

5 SIGNS TO LOOK OUT FOR

If you are striving to keep yourself healthy for now and many years to come, and you want to know what single thing you should be paying attention to more than anything else, it is this: inflammation.

The reason inflammation is so critical is that it has been found to be a player in almost every chronic disease. And if it hasn't been shown to be associated with a chronic disease, it's probably just because no one has looked for it.

You probably wouldn't be surprised to hear that it is a major part of autoimmune diseases since they are all directly caused by the immune system. Maybe you've also already heard that the white cells that sneak into the walls of your arteries are major contributors to cardiovascular disease, meaning it's not just about cholesterol build-up. Perhaps you also know that cancer tends to form in areas that are chronically inflamed. But you might not have expected inflammation to be a component of osteoarthritis, the disease that we doctors thought was just from too much tackle football or tennis (wear and tear of the bones). Inflammation even plays a role in hypertension and depression.

Top 5 Symptoms of Chronic Inflammation

At Parsley Health, one of our main goals is to help people prevent and reverse chronic disease, so we pay a lot of attention to chronic inflammation. We look for symptoms of inflammation beginning at our patients' very first visit. Here are five common indications that someone may have a chronic inflammatory condition:

Body pain, especially in the joints

Skin rashes, such as eczema or psoriasis

Excessive mucus production (ie, always needing to clear your throat or blow your nose)

Low energy, despite sufficient sleep

Poor digestion, including bloating, abdominal pain, constipation and loose stool

We're diving deep into inflammation. Get our newsletter to read every piece as it's published.

The Tests Your Doctor Should Be Doing

Not only do we listen for inflammation in our patients' histories, but we also test for it in every patient we see using these three biomarkers:

White blood cell count

Sedimentation rate (ESR)

High sensitivity c-reactive protein (hsCRP). (Note: About 1/3 of the adult U.S. population has an elevated CRP.)

Each one of these looks at different components of the blood to see if there is inflammation in the body. They are non-specific, meaning they don't tell us where the inflammation is coming from, but they do clue us in to look harder for it. Taken together, we get a pretty good idea as to whether inflammation is an issue, and we can also use them to track if the inflammation is resolving or worsening.

160

How to Heal Chronic Inflammation

If all this talk of chronic inflammation and its pervasive effect on chronic disease is getting you nervous, don't worry! You actually don't need to know which cytokine blocks which receptor to know what to do.

Our recommended approach is very similar to what we recommend for health in general:

Remove the foods that are known to cause inflammation, like sugar, dairy and simple carbohydrates.

Avoid foods that you are sensitive to. This is something we often test for or figure out with an elimination diet.

Eat lots of foods that are known to be anti-inflammatory, like leafy greens, colorful veggies, nuts, seeds, herbs and spices (eg, turmeric, ginger and rosemary) and extra virgin olive oil.

Exercise. Regular exercise of moderate intensity improves immune function and decreases inflammation.(Even occasional exercise has benefits, but high-intensity exercise may actually have a detrimental effect on the immune system.)

Minimize stress and optimize how you respond to it.

Supplements such as probiotics, turmeric, resveratrol and fish oil are known to help fight inflammation.

Inflammation is an amazing unifier of most chronic diseases, so if you want to optimize your current and future health, you can do so by minimizing inflammation. Take note if you have symptoms that seem consistent with inflammation, check for it with blood tests, and do your best to adopt an anti-inflammatory lifestyle.

Ways To Reduce Inflammation

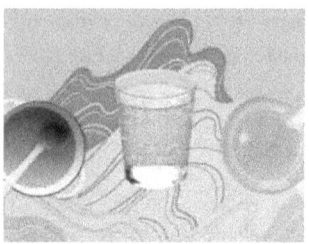

I started connecting the dots between my diet and lifestyle, chronic inflammation, and disease, a light bulb turned on. Why? Because our daily choices are at the root of chronic inflammation.

Over the past decade, I've renovated everything from my grocery cart to my makeup bag to my mind in an effort to upgrade my immune system. And as I moved from a stressful life full of fast food, toxins, and bad boyfriends to a more balanced existence filled with plant-passionate nourishment, inner growth, and conscious living, I started experiencing the perks. Chronic inflammation decreased and my body started working with me to heal and rebuild.

Want to start connecting the dots in your own life? First, let's learn about acute and chronic inflammation, since they play very different roles in our everyday health. Then, we'll cover the causes of chronic inflammation and how to reduce its impact on your health.

The Results of Chronic Inflammation

Over time, chronic inflammation wears out your immune system, leading to chronic diseases and other health issues including cancer, asthma, autoimmune diseases, allergies, irritable bowel syndrome, arthritis, osteoporosis, and even (gasp!) appearing older than your years.

Unfortunately, these challenges are often only treated with drugs and surgery, which may provide temporary relief from the symptoms, but do not treat the root of the problem. In addition, these drugs and their side effects sometimes only add to your health problems.

Could it be that many of the pills in your cabinet are just Band-Aids and that the key to health lies in your daily diet and lifestyle choices? That's certainly what I've found to be true.

The integrative MDs I know and trust are helping their patients identify and address their health issues by looking at the way they lead their lives and nipping their inflammation-happy habits in the bud. If possible, find an integrative doctor who can help you along the way and target your unique needs. They can also test your blood for inflammation make sure your doc requests a CRP—C-reactive Protein test.

Although this may seem overwhelming, it's actually the opposite. The following tips will empower you and help you reduce inflammation over time. Try a few (or just one) of these suggestions on for size and see how you feel. As always, slow and steady wins the race, or in this case, puts out the fire.

How to Reduce Chronic Inflammation

4. Eat more plant-based, whole, nutrient-dense foods.

Crowd out the inflammatory foods we discussed above (refined sugar and flour, processed junk, animal products, etc.) by adding a variety of plant-based whole foods to your diet. These foods will flood your body with the vitamins, minerals, cancer-fighting phytochemicals, antioxidants, and fiber it needs to recover from chronic inflammation.

5. Focus on gut health.

Your gut holds approximately 60 to 70 percent of your immune system, so it stands to reason that it would be a great place to reduce chronic inflammation. And if your gut is in bad shape, you can only imagine that your immune system is in some serious trouble. Check out my tips for improving gut health here. A great way to start is by taking a daily probiotic.

6. Identify and address food allergies and chronic (or hidden) infections.

You could be fighting a losing battle if you're ignoring potential food sensitivities and/or infections. If your body is working to cope and fight these challenges every day, you can bet that you're stoking the fires of inflammation on a regular basis.

Gluten, soy, dairy, eggs, and yeast are common food allergens that might be distracting your immune system every time you sit down for a meal. These allergies can be identified with a blood test. Ask your doctor about testing for food allergies.

Become a symptoms detective. Only you can determine how you feel when you eat, which is where an elimination diet comes in handy. While following the elimination approach, you remove all common allergens from your diet and then slowly reintroduce them, one by one. Talk to your doc about these options, and do some independent research at Google University.

Another possibility worth exploring is chronic infection (bacteria, viruses, yeast, parasites). These guys could be hiding out in your body just under the radar and dragging your immune system down. You have a couple options for testing—look at your bloodwork and/or your poop. It may not be pretty, but knowledge is power, so be brave and have your stool checked. You can have your stool analyzed—this analysis will identify parasites, abnormal bacteria, yeasts, and other gastrointestinal issues, which will help you create a game plan that targets the infection, ideally with the help of an integrative MD or naturopath.

You may also want to look into Leaky Gut Syndrome, a condition that can result in damage to your intestinal lining. When this occurs, bacteria, undigested food, and other toxins can literally leak into your bloodstream, triggering an autoimmune response and a host of painful inflammatory symptoms. A simple urine test can tell you if you need to plug up those leaks, so to speak.

7. Relax and rest more.

Your body is hard at work repairing and restoring your glorious cells while you sleep. Most doctors recommend 7 to 8 hours of sleep per night. If you're cutting corners in the snooze department, you're cheating your immune system, which means it needs to kick into high gear in an effort to keep you well (hello, inflammation).

Stress goes hand in hand with a lack of sleep and a laundry list of demands from daily life. Unfortunately, when you're stressed out all the time, you're also producing more of the hormone cortisol inflammation's BFF. It stands to reason that you can easily reduce chronic inflammation by focusing on stress reduction, whether it's through more sleep, yoga, meditation, long walks, less technology, or a much-needed vacation. You know I love to take every opportunity I can to remind you to take a chill pill.

8. Reduce toxins in your food, home, and personal care products.

Your body's alarm system goes off when you absorb toxic chemicals and pesticides through your digestive tract and your skin. Cut down your exposure by eating organic foods whenever possible and choosing non-toxic personal care and cleaning products.

THE FUNGUS ANTI-INFLAMMATORY DIET AND HOW IT MAY TREAT YOUR NAIL FUNGUS

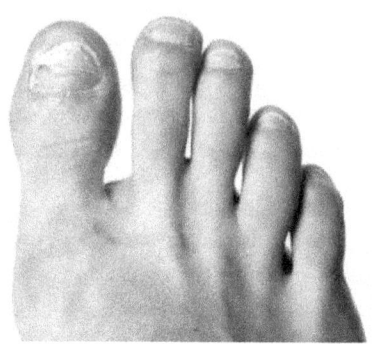

What is nail fungus?

The anti-inflammatory diet can help boost your immune system, which can help fight off fungal infections. Drinking the recommended six to eight glasses of water a day is suggested with this diet, which can help to cleanse your inner system, also helping to fight off infection.

In addition to being helpful in the fight to rid oneself of a fungus infection, there are other health benefits attached to the diet such as help with depression and improved mental state, a stronger immune system, less water retainage and more.

What is the Anti-Inflammatory Diet?

The anti-inflammatory diet usually consists of eating 2,000 to 3,000 calories a day. The amount of calories depends on your size. You should be eating 40 to 50% of carbohydrates, 30 % of fat and include carbohydrates, fat and protein with each meal.

This diet uses a lot of fish and fresh fruits and vegetables while minimizing the consumption of fast food meals. Beans, winter squashes and sweet potatoes are also a big part of this diet.

This diet is not typically meant for weight loss, but can be used for health reasons and is said to help with fungal problems.

How do I know if it's working?

It may take a little while for the diet to work. Remember, if you've been eating a totally different diet, particularly if it was a poor diet, it will take a while for your system to be completely cleaned out. You might want to make a visit to a nutritionist or to the local health food store to discuss how and when the diet will work.

You can expect any treatment to take six to twelve weeks to work and the change in your diet alone may not be enough. Keep a journal of what you eat and do and any changes you see if you are unsure of the effectiveness of treatment.

Okay, I'm on the diet, what else should I be doing?

Again, this is something to be discussed with your healthcare physician, a dietitian or nutritionist or even your health foot store representative who is well-versed in dietary needs. At times, a health foot store may have different or more reliable information than the internet or even your physician's office and may be able to give you some supplements, topical creams or organic lacquers which may prove to be extremely effective, especially in conjunction with the anti-inflammatory diet.

You may also want to check your library or local book store. Internet research can be helpful when making a decision regarding informational books on nail fungus and diet-related and other organic treatment remedies.

THE EASIEST CHANGES TO BOOST HEALTH

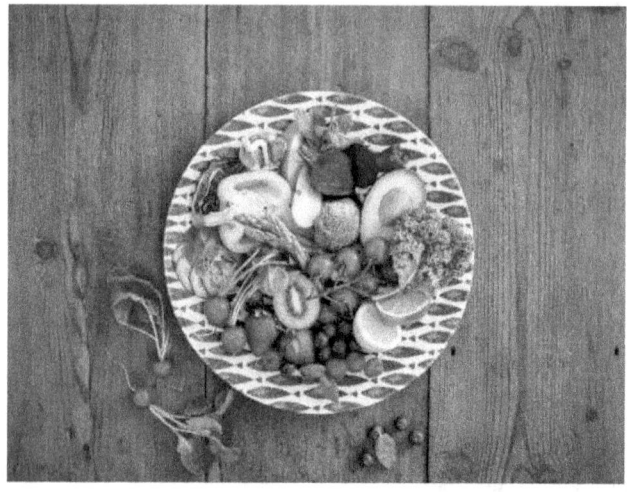

There are a million and one trendy diets out there offering to change how you look and feel in a matter of days. The consumer is flooded with products that will make their skin "appear" healthier and softer to touch. In a world with too much focus on looking good and "appearing" healthier, there is one diet that WILL make you healthier and potentially live a longer life in your anti-aged body.

The anti-inflammatory diet has so many uses today it is surprising every one of the health, fitness and beauty gurus have not jumped on the simplest of diet changes and marketed them as the next big trend in weight loss, beauty and anti-aging. The fact is the anti-inflammatory diet can do everything other diets claim they can do and increase lifespan in the process.

So how do I jump start the anti-inflammatory diet?

Think of this first week as a natural eating time, so don't make any changes or eat anything you would not normally eat. Once the list is complete, head off to the Internet for a little research and education on the power of food over inflammation. Many people are surprised by the effects seemingly healthy foods can have on overall body health and the prevention of illness. Sure, the market screams at the consumer about drinking more vitamin C and reducing calories, but what about the foods that seem healthy but really aren't? These foods will be found after a week of journaling before starting your anti-inflammatory diet.

Are there any baked foods on the list? Chances are, if these foods were purchased prepackaged; they will contain at least a small amount of trans fats. Even the small, 100 calorie bites of cupcake marketed as healthy alternatives can contain up to 0.5 grams of trans fats. Eating just two of these little cakes a day for a week contributes a whopping 7 grams of trans fats - the only healthy level is 0 grams.

Did you eat a salad this week? Many people think eating a salad is a healthy alternative and it can be, without that fat laden dressing covering the healthy greens. One tablespoon of regular dressing can contain 100 calories and about 10 grams of fat. The typical true serving is about ¼ cup per salad. That equates to 400 calories, 40 grams of fat and a -76 rating on the inflammation factor scale which measures the total inflammatory effect of foods on the body.

EATING ANTI-INFLAMMATORY FOODS

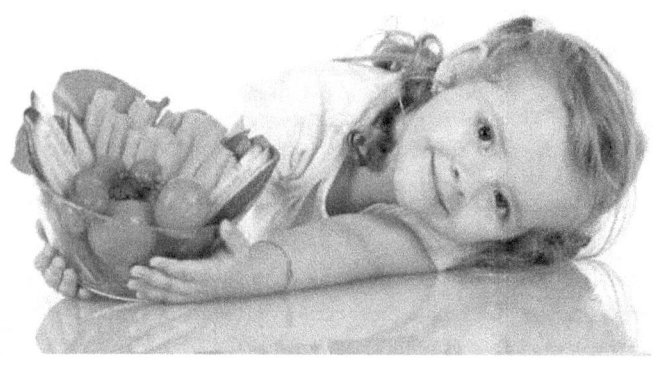

Are there really diets out there that can reduce inflammation? Do they work? Scientists have found that there is a relationship, in part, between what we eat and inflammation. They've even identified some compounds in food that can reduce inflammation and others that promote it. There is still a lot to learn about just how diet and inflammation interact, and research, as of yet, is not at that point where a specific foods or groups of foods can be singled out as being beneficial for people with arthritis. We are beginning to get a clearer picture of how eating the right way can reduce inflammation.

So why are we so concerned about inflammation? Inflammation is the body's natural defense to infections and injuries. When something goes wrong the body's immune system goes to work to inflame the area, which serves to get rid of the invader or to heal the wound. Inflammation can cause pain, swelling, redness, and warmth, but this goes away as soon as the problem is solved. This is good inflammation.

Then we have chronic inflammation, the type that's familiar to people with rheumatoid arthritis (RA), lupus, psoriatic arthritis, and other types of "inflammatory" arthritis.

Chronic inflammation is the type that will not go away. All the types of arthritis that are mentioned above are a disorder of the immune system creates inflammation and then doesn't know when to shut off. Inflammatory arthritis, chronic inflammation can have serious consequences, permanent disability and tissue damage can be one if it isn't treated properly. Inflammation has been linked to a full host of other medical conditions.

Inflammation has been found to contribute to atherosclerosis, which is when fat builds up on the lining of arteries, raising the risk of heart attacks. Also, high levels of inflammation proteins have been found in the blood of people with heart disease. Inflammation has also been linked to obesity, diabetes, asthma, depression, and even Alzheimer disease and cancer. Scientists think that a constant level of inflammation in the body, even if the level is low, can have a number of negative effects. Research shows that diet can reduce inflammation; in theory an inflammation-lowering diet should have an effect on a wide range of health conditions.

Researchers have looked for clues in the eating habits of our early ancestors to discover which foods might benefit us the most. They believe those habits are more in tune to our eating habits with how the body processes and uses what we eat and drink. Our ancestor's diet consisted of wild lean meats (venison or boar) and wild plants (green leafy vegetables, fruits, nuts, and berries). There were no cereal grains until the agriculture revolution (about 10,000 years ago). There was very little dairy, and there were no processed or refined foods. Our diets are usually are high in meat, saturated (or bad) fats, and processed foods, and there is very little exercise. Nearly everything we eat is available close by or as far away as our computer and the click of a mouse.

Our diet and lifestyles are way out of whack with how our bodies are made from the inside out. While our genetic make-up has changed very little from our early beginnings, our diet and lifestyles have changed a great deal and the changes have gotten worse over the last 50 to 100 years. Our genes haven't had a chance to adapt. We aren't giving our bodies the right kind of fuel, it's as though we think of our bodies as engines in a jet plane when instead they are like the engine in the very first planes. There are some foods that we are putting into our bodies, especially because we are eating way too much of them, that are affecting our health in a bad way.

There are two nutrients in our diets that have attracted attention, are omega-3 fatty acids and omega-6 fatty acids have been part of our diets for thousands of years. They are components in just about all of our many cells and are important for normal growth and development. Both of these acids play a role in inflammation. In several studies it was found that certain sources of omega 3's in particular, help to reduce the inflammation process and that omega 6's will raise it.

Now this is the problem, the average American eats on average about 15 times more omega 6's than omega 3's. While our very early ancestor's ate omega 6's and omega 3's in equal ratio, and it is believed that this is what helped to balance their ability to turn inflammation on and off. The imbalance of omega 3's and omega 6's in our diets is believed to contribute to the excess of inflammation in our bodies.

So why is it that we eat so many omega 6's now? Vegetable oils such as corn oil, safflower oil, sunflower oil, cottonseed oil, soybean oil, and the products made from them, such as margarine, are loaded with omega 6's. Even many of the processed snack foods that are so readily available today are full of these oils. Based on the best information of the time, was to use vegetable oils like those mentioned above instead of foods with saturated fats such as butter and lard. It looks like the consequences of that advice may have contributed to the increased consumption of omega 6's and therefore causing an imbalance of omega 3's and omega 6's.

You can find omega 6's in other common foods such as meats and egg yolks. The omega 6 found in meat is the fatty acids that come from grain-fed animals such as cows, lambs, pigs and chickens. Most of the meat sold in America is grain fed unlike their grass-fed cousins who contain less of those fatty acids. Wild game such as venison and boar are lower in omega 6's and fat and higher in omega 3's than the meat that comes from the supermarkets where we shop.

You can get omega 3s in both animal and plant food. Our bodies can convert omega 3s from animal sources into anti-inflammatory compounds more easily than the omega 3s from plant sources. Plant foods contain hundreds of other healthful compounds many of which that are anti-inflammatory, so don't discount them all together.

There are many foods that are high in omega 3s and that include fatty fish, especially fish from cold waters. Of course everyone knows about salmon but did you know that you can also find omega 3s in mackerel, anchovies, sardines, herring, striped bass, and bluefish. It's also widely known that wild fish are better sources of omega 3s than the farm raised ones. You can also buy eggs that have been enriched with omega 3 oils. There are several excellent sources of omega 3s in plants that are leafy greens (like kale, Swiss chard, and spinach) as well as flaxseed, wheat germ, walnuts, and their oils.

You can also get omega 3s in supplements (often as fish oil); this source has been shown to be beneficial in some instances. You should take with your doctor before you take a fish oil supplement because it can interact with some medications and under certain circumstances can increase the risk of bleeding. I take a prescribed omega 3 supplement because my doctor had told me that the ones you get in the supermarket or health food store are not pure, they have other additives that do absolutely nothing to help. There are other fats that are contributors to clogged arteries, the "bad" or saturated fats found in meats and high-fat dairy foods, these are called pro-inflammatory.

There are also the Trans fats that are relatively new to the cause of heart disease. These Trans fats can be found in processed convenience and snack foods and can be spotted by reading the labels. They can be identified as partially hydrogenated oils, often soybean oil or cottonseed oil. But, they can also occur naturally in small amounts in animal foods. The thought is that they contribute to the pro-inflammatory activities in our bodies and the amounts we eat today are staggering.

Antioxidants are substances that prevent inflammation causing "free radicals" from over taking our bodies. Plant foods such as fruits, vegetables (including beans), nuts, and seeds carry high amounts of antioxidants. Extra-virgin olive oil and walnut oil are very good sources of antioxidants, also. These foods have long been considered the basics for good health, and can be found in fruits and vegetables with colorful and vibrant pigments. The more colorful the plant, the better they are for you, from green vegetables, especially leafy ones, to low-starch vegetables, such as broccoli and cauliflower, to berries, tomatoes, and brightly colored orange and yellow fruits and vegetables.

I bet you're wondering what this has to do with Arthritis. Well, there has been some research on diet and arthritis, mostly focusing on RA. There was a study that looked into a bunch of other studies on diet and RA and found that diets high in omega 3's had some effect on reducing the symptoms of RA. There was yet another study published in 2008, that found eating omega 6 fatty acids and omega 3 fatty acids in a ratio of 2 or 3 to 1 (a low ratio compared to the 15 to 1 ratio in most people's diet) decreased the inflammation in people with RA. There was also another study that found taking omega 3 may also allow people to reduce their use of no steroidal anti-inflammatory drugs (NSAIDs), such as ibuprofen (Advil, Motrin) and naproxen (Aleve). But these and other studies don't offer enough evidence to prove that there is any particular anti-inflammatory diet that can have a real impact on arthritis symptoms. It doesn't mean that the diets are harmful; it just means that there may come a day when research may be able to prove their benefits. In the future, diet may be considered one of the many tools along with exercise and medicine that can be used to ease the symptoms of arthritis.

We don't have to revert back completely to the caveman to eat the anti-inflammatory way to benefit from the anti-inflammatory diet. Just eating a healthful diet that is recommended today is right on track. Our chief strategy should be to balance the amount of modern day foods with the foods of long ago, which were rich in the inflammation reducing foods. Really, all we have to do is replace foods rich in omega 6 with foods rich in omega 3, cutting down on how much meat and poultry we eat while eating oily fish a couple of times a week and adding more varieties of colorful fruits and vegetables, and while whole grains were not a part of our early ancestor's diet, it should be included in ours. Be sure that it is whole grains and not refined grains because they contain many beneficial nutrients and inflammation-tempering compounds. Researchers have found that eating a lot of foods high in sugar and white flour may promote inflammation, although there is more studying that needs to be done on the subject.

The amounts of knowledge we have on how the body works and how our ancestor's ate is helping to confirm the old adage: "You are what you eat." But, there is still more we need to learn before we can prescribe any one anti-inflammatory diet. Our genetic makeup and the severity of our health condition will determine the benefits we get from an anti-inflammatory diet and unfortunately there is doubt that there will be one diet that fits us all.

Also, what we eat or don't eat is just a small part of the whole story. We are not as physically active as our ancestors and physical activity has its own anti-inflammatory effects. Our ancestors were also much leaner than we are and body fat is active tissue that can make inflammatory producing compounds.

Anti-inflammatory eating is a way of selecting foods that are more in tune with what the body actually needs. We can achieve a more balanced diet by going back to our roots. If you look at the diet of the people of the Bible, you will find that they, like our caveman ancestors, were more active and their diets consisted of much the same things as our caveman ancestors. They also had no choice but to walk everywhere they wanted to go, there was no such thing as cars or trucks. While we have it easier today, our health has suffered greatly from it.

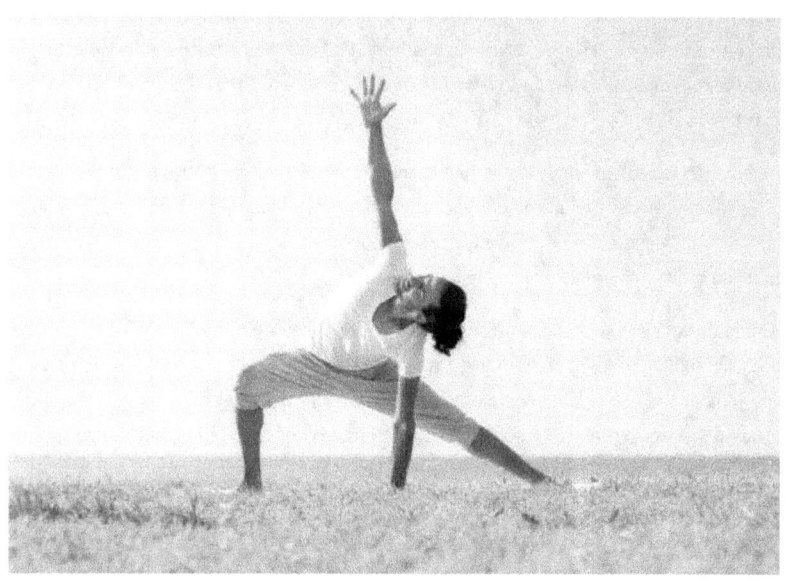

Your immune system becomes activated when your body recognizes anything that is foreign such as an invading microbe, plant pollen, or chemical. This often triggers a process called inflammation. Intermittent bouts of inflammation directed at truly threatening invaders protect your health.

However, sometimes inflammation persists, day in and day out, even when you are not threatened by a foreign invader. That's when inflammation can become your enemy. Many major diseases that plague us including cancer, heart disease, diabetes, arthritis, depression, and Alzheimer's have been linked to chronic inflammation.

Choose the right anti-inflammatory foods, and you may be able to reduce your risk of illness. Consistently pick the wrong ones, and you could accelerate the inflammatory disease process.

Foods that cause inflammation

Try to avoid or limit these foods as much as possible:

refined carbohydrates, such as white bread and pastries

French fries and other fried foods

soda and other sugar-sweetened beverages

red meat (burgers, steaks) and processed meat (hot dogs, sausage)

margarine, shortening, and lard.

The health risks of inflammatory foods

Not surprisingly, the same foods on an inflammation diet are generally considered bad for our health, including sodas and refined carbohydrates, as well as red meat and processed meats.

"Some of the foods that have been associated with an increased risk for chronic diseases such as type 2 diabetes and heart disease are also associated with excess inflammation. "It's not surprising, since inflammation is an important underlying mechanism for the development of these diseases."

Unhealthy foods also contribute to weight gain, which is itself a risk factor for inflammation. Yet in several studies, even after researchers took obesity into account, the link between foods and inflammation remained, which suggests weight gain isn't the sole driver. "Some of the food components or ingredients may have independent effects on inflammation over and above increased caloric intake,

Anti-inflammatory foods

An anti-inflammatory diet should include these foods:

tomatoes

olive oil

green leafy vegetables, such as spinach, kale, and collards

nuts like almonds and walnuts

fatty fish like salmon, mackerel, tuna, and sardines

fruits such as strawberries, blueberries, cherries, and oranges

Benefits of anti-inflammatory foods

On the flip side are beverages and foods that reduce inflammation, and with it, chronic disease, He notes in particular fruits and vegetables such as blueberries, apples, and leafy greens that are high in natural antioxidants and polyphenols—protective compounds found in plants.

Studies have also associated nuts with reduced markers of inflammation and a lower risk of cardiovascular disease and diabetes. Coffee, which contains polyphenols and other anti-inflammatory compounds, may protect against inflammation, as well.

Anti-inflammatory diet

To reduce levels of inflammation, aim for an overall healthy diet. If you're looking for an eating plan that closely follows the tenets of anti-inflammatory eating, consider the Mediterranean diet, which is high in fruits, vegetables, nuts, whole grains, fish, and healthy oils.

In addition to lowering inflammation, a more natural, less processed diet can have noticeable effects on your physical and emotional health

The Benefits of an Anti-Inflammatory Diet

One of the most common problems I address with patients involves the treatment of chronic pain. The day-to-day aches and pains that make life sometimes unbearable. Many people feel that being given drugs for the pain is not the answer, and they seek natural remedies instead.

What Causes Pain

One of the most common causes of pain is chronic inflammation. Inflammation can be described as a condition whereby our tissues become irritated due to injury or infection. The symptoms of inflammation include pain, swelling, red discoloration, heat, stiffness, and/or limited range of motion. There are several conditions that can cause chronic inflammation, including autoimmune conditions like Crohn's disease and rheumatoid arthritis. Chronic inflammation has also been thought to be a contributing factor to conditions like Alzheimer's disease and certain types of heart disease.

Avoid Foods that Cause Inflammation

One of the first things you can do to reduce chronic inflammation is to consider removing foods from your diet that are thought to cause inflammation. The most inflammatory foods are the foods with the highest risk of sensitivity and allergy. The most common food allergies and pro-inflammatory foods are mentioned below.

8. Milk and all dairy products (yogurt, cheese, butter, etc.) not only contain lactose, a sugar many people cannot digest, but a substance called casein. Casein is a protein found in dairy products, and can be pro-inflammatory in many people.

9. Wheat and all wheat products (pasta, bread, cookies, cake, etc.) can be very inflammatory in many people. This is because many people are sensitive to products that contain gluten. If you have not been tested for gluten sensitivity or allergy, try giving up wheat products for 6 to 8 weeks and then reintroducing them. If you feel better off without wheat products and worse on them, this might be a sign of gluten sensitivity. (Please note today that there are many kosher products available on the market that are gluten-free.)

10. Eggs, which can also be found in cakes, sauces, protein powders and many baked goods. Some people are allergic to either the egg whites, the egg yolks, or both. Again, if you have not been tested for food sensitivities, try giving this food up for 6 to 8 weeks and reintroducing it to see if you have a reaction.

11. Meat that is not organic but advertised as corn-fed or vegetarian-fed. If you are looking for kosher organic meat, it does exist, and can be found in some health food stores—try first checking online, or going to your local health food store to find out if they can start carrying it. The reason inorganic meat is pro-inflammatory is because it contains high amounts of a substance called arachidonic acid. Arachidonic acid is a substance found in our cells that initiates something called the PGE2 pathway. This is the process by which a cell undergoes inflammation. Thus, it is believed that too much arachidonic acid in the diet can trigger inflammation.

12. All overly processed foods that contain corn syrup and sugar, like candy bars and soda pops, and processed and cured meats, like hot dogs and sausages.

13.   Nightshade vegetables, which include potatoes, tomatoes, and eggplants. These foods contain a substance called solanine, which has been found to cause pain and inflammation in some people.

14.   Some people may also be sensitive to citrus fruits like oranges, as well as some tropical fruits like papayas, mangos and pineapples.

What Can I Eat on an Anti-Inflammatory Diet?

5. Try to eat fruits and vegetables that are locally grown, organic and in season. You may want to start looking into buying your produce from local farmers' markets, where produce is often the freshest.

6. Eat meat sparingly, and whenever possible choose meat that is organic. Many companies are now producing organic kosher meats. Lean meats like chicken, turkey and fish are best. Please click here for more information on organic kosher meat.

7. Try to eat cold-water fish and smaller fish. They tend to contain the least amount of mercury and the highest amounts of omega-3 fatty acids, which have anti-inflammatory benefits.

8. Begin to add spices found to decrease inflammation like turmeric. Other spices that decrease inflammation include ginger and rosemary.

9. Begin incorporating whole organic beans and whole grains into your diet. There are many delicious stews and soups with which you can begin to experiment, that use many grains with which you might not be familiar. This include quinoa, brown rice, millet, and unbleached barley, to name a few. Whole grains and beans also offer us a wide variety of nutrients and fiber. Fiber has the added benefit of aiding in healthy digestion. Fiber can also be helpful in lowering cholesterol.

10. Try to choose oils that are cold pressed, like olive oil. These oils are less processed and, unlike margarine, are not solid at room temperature. They are less inflammatory then the hydrogenated oils, like margarine, and are better for the health of the heart.

While some of these changes may be challenging to incorporate into your diet at first, you will find that they can be quite helpful in reducing inflammation and chronic pain, and can help improve your overall health as well.

KEYS TO REDUCING INFLAMMATION

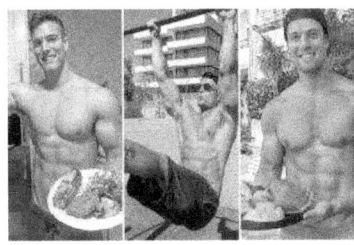

Inflammation (swelling), which is part of the body's natural healing system, helps fight injury and infection. But it doesn't just happen in response to injury and illness.

An inflammatory response can also occur when the immune system goes into action without an injury or infection to fight. Since there's nothing to heal, the immune system cells that normally protect us begin to destroy healthy arteries, organs and joints.

What does chronic inflammation do to the body?

Early symptoms of chronic inflammation may be vague, with subtle signs and symptoms that may go undetected for a long period. You may just feel slightly fatigued, or even normal. As inflammation progresses, however, it begins to damage your arteries, organs and joints. Left unchecked, it can contribute to chronic diseases, such as heart disease, blood vessel disease, diabetes, obesity, cancer, Alzheimer's disease and other conditions.

Immune system cells that cause inflammation contribute to the buildup of fatty deposits in the lining of the heart's arteries. These plaques can eventually rupture, which causes a clot to form that could potentially block an artery. When blockage happens, the result is a heart attack.

What can I do to reduce the risk of chronic inflammation?

You can control and even reverse inflammation through a healthy, anti-inflammatory lifestyle. People with a family history of health problems, such as heart disease or colon cancer, should talk to their physicians about lifestyle changes that support preventing disease by reducing inflammation.

Follow these six tips for reducing inflammation in your body:

5. Load up on anti-inflammatory foods

Your food choices are just as important as the medications and supplements you may be taking for overall health since they can protect against inflammation. "An anti-inflammatory diet emphasizes foods that reduce inflammation.

Eat more fruits and vegetables and foods containing omega-3 fatty acids. Some of the best sources of omega-3s are cold water fish, such as salmon and tuna, and tofu, walnuts, flax seeds and soybeans.

Other anti-inflammatory foods include grapes, celery, blueberries, garlic, olive oil, tea and some spices (ginger, rosemary and turmeric).

The Mediterranean diet is an example of an anti-inflammatory diet. This is due to its focus on fruits, vegetables, fish and whole grains, and limits on unhealthy fats, such as red meat, butter and egg yolks as well as processed and refined sugars and carbs.

6. Cut back or eliminate inflammatory foods

Inflammatory foods include red meat and anything with trans fats, such as margarine, corn oil, deep fried foods and most processed foods.

7. Control blood sugar

Limit or avoid simple carbohydrates, such as white flour, white rice, refined sugar and anything with high fructose corn syrup.

One easy rule to follow is to avoid white foods, such as white bread, rice and pasta, as well as foods made with white sugar and flour. Build meals around lean proteins and whole foods high in fiber, such as vegetables, fruits and whole grains, such as brown rice and whole wheat bread. Check the labels and make sure that "whole wheat" or another whole grain is the first ingredient.

8. Make time to exercise

Make time for 30 to 45 minutes of aerobic exercise and 10 to 25 minutes of weight or resistance training at least four to five times per week.

9. Lose weight

People who are overweight have more inflammation. Losing weight may decrease inflammation.

10.   Manage stress

Chronic stress contributes to inflammation. Use meditation, yoga, biofeedback, guided imagery or some other method to manage stress throughout the day.

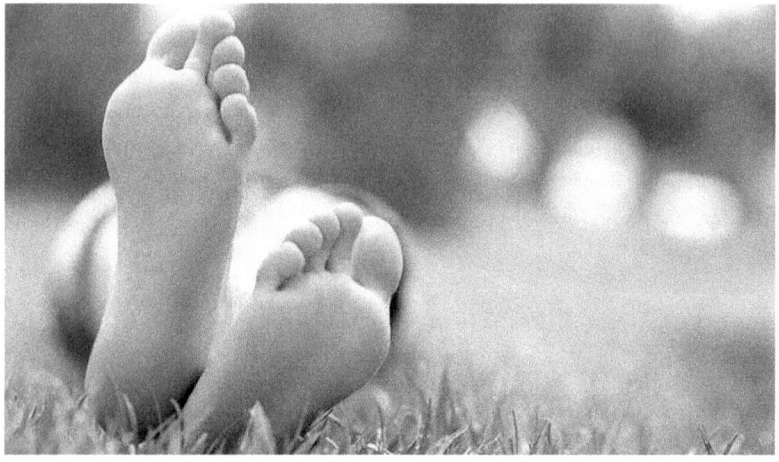

Inflammation is often associated with injury. You stub your toe and the toe swells. This is the basic inflammatory reaction. Some people even understand that redness around a cut is also a form of inflammation that the immune system uses to heal the injury. What is not commonly known is the fact that inflammation occurs inside the body as well. When the body exists in an inflammatory state, risk of illness, cancer and heart conditions can increase. An anti-inflammatory diet is an easy way to combat this aftereffect and reduce risk today.

I Don't Suffer From Inflammation!

This is the most common statement and the least correct. Inflammation affects every person in the world at some point in their life. In western cultures, like the United States, a huge portion of the population is affected by inflammation every day. Being overweight or obese is the most common inflammatory condition. It is this inflammatory response that could be the cause of some weight related conditions like diabetes.

When fat cells grow, they take up the free space around the organs. Blood flow can be constricted and the body often feels as though it needs to fight to function normally. When the body feels threatened, inflammation occurs as a natural, healing response. Unfortunately, unlike the small cut that will heal in a few, short days. Obesity takes time to correct and the longer the body lives inflamed, the greater the risk of long term effects.

In the case of obesity, changing the diet by reducing calories will reduce body weight and thus reduce the inflammation in the body. This is the simplest benefit of an anti-inflammatory diet. However, people who are obese or overweight are not the only people who can benefit from an anti-inflammatory diet.

Illness Treatment and Prevention

There are many illnesses and conditions caused by inflammation. These include asthma, arthritis, inflammatory bowel syndrome, pelvic inflammatory disease, endometriosis, diabetes, COPD, Psoriasis, Colitis, and Lupus - just to name a few. All-in-all, there are nearly 40 autoimmune conditions currently accepted by the medical community that are affected by inflammation.

What Can I Do?

The first step is to make dietary changes to reduce food based inflammation. Processed foods, fast foods and prepackaged foods can cause increased inflammation in the body. Replacing these foods with lean meats, whole grains and healthy fats will make a tremendous different in how the body reacts to inflammation. In addition, if weight is a problem, reducing weight while changing to an anti-inflammatory diet can increase the benefits exponentially.

Changing to an anti-inflammatory diet does not have to be in reaction to a disease or illness. Prevention is the best choice and the anti-inflammatory diet can reduce the risk of contracting many of the listed illnesses. When the body feels as though it needs to fight for survival, inflammation occurs, so offering healthy foods that have an inflammatory effect is a great choice for all people including those who are young, healthy and feel they do not need an anti-inflammatory diet.

STRUGGLES OF AN ANTI-INFLAMMATORY DIET

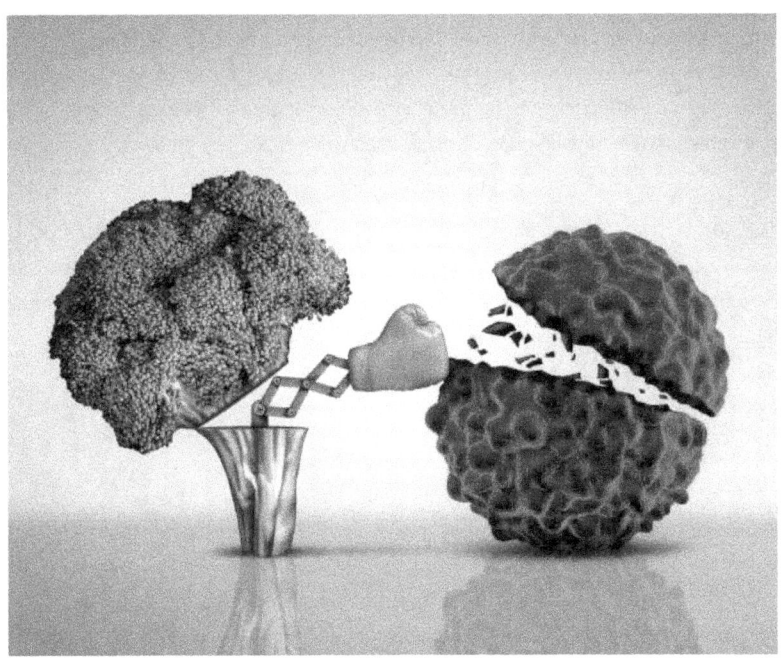

Everyone wants to feel better and live in better health. One of the easiest ways to achieve that is by switching from a traditional western diet to an anti-inflammatory diet. Making the change is easy, but much like a diet plan, sticking with the food changes and watching what you eat can be difficult.

Fast Food and Your Inflammation

Fast food is a huge hindrance to the anti-inflammatory diet. Foods that are high in fat tend to increase inflammatory substances in the body for three to four hours after the meal. If the same number of calories eaten in one fast food sitting were eaten as fresh fruits, vegetables and lean meats, this effect would not occur. Free radicals, cell killers that compound inflammation problems, can also be increased by 175% after eating fast food.

The Alternative - The best alternative to fast food is a replacement, anti-inflammatory diet. This sandwich can be made from lean ground turkey and a whole grain bun. The "special" sauce can be mixed up with lower carbohydrate ketchup, olive oil mayonnaise and sugar free relish. The result is a tasty alternative with a significantly lower fat count.

Red Meat, Milk and Your Inflammation

Science has long fought to connect red meat with certain forms of cancer. Little did they know the research would lead to a link between this common dinner protein and inflammation. Researchers believe the body reacts to certain chemical aspects of red meat and milk in a protective manner. If the body believes these are foreign substances, the immune system will kick in and inflammation occurs. Imagine eating red meat once a day and drinking two or three glasses of milk. The body would live in a state of constant or chronic inflammation which could cause health problems over time.

The Alternative - Lean poultry, beef and fish are all part of a healthy diet. Beef is a great source of iron, so eliminating it is not a necessity. But, choosing the leanest of cuts is essential to good health. The best meats are lean proteins and beans.

Trans Fats and Your Inflammation

A hidden source of body inflammation is the trans fatty acid. While many people know a bit about this type of fat, few understand the effects on the body. Fast food, baked goods, prepackaged meals and margarine are often good sources of trans fat. After entering the body, these fats can increase the risk of coronary artery disease, insulin resistance, diabetes and heart failure. Increased risk of stroke due to abnormally high lipid levels is also common. While many foods will claim to be trans fat free, that is not the entire truth. According to labeling guidelines, these foods can contain up to 0.5 grams of trans fats per serving and still mark the product as "trans fat free". These small amounts will add up over time if the diet is rich in processed foods, margarine and baked goods.

The Alternative - Natural fats like whole butter and olive oil have no trans fats. Choosing these in place of hydrogenated oils and margarine is a good first step. When it comes to foods cooked in trans fat, there is no choice but to eliminate these from the diet all together.

The Anti-Inflammatory Diet for Arthritis Relief

Food and arthritis have a connection to each other and that is why changing your diet is one of the first pieces of advice an expert can give a person with inflammation in his or her joints. There are foods that can reduce inflammation and there are those that might worsen the inflammation. A person with arthritis should follow the anti-inflammatory diet if he or she wants to get treated. To start an anti-inflammatory diet, one should know which foods he or she going to eliminate in one's diet and which foods will be added.

What are the foods that you should avoid and eliminate in your diet? When it comes to arthritis, it is always advised that the person affected should eliminate artificial foods like junk foods, those foods that have been processed and foods with added artificial flavorings and colorings. A person with arthritis should also avoid meats that have high levels of fats and foods that are high in sugar. The reasons why these kinds of foods should be avoided by people with arthritis is that the saturated fats and trans fats found in these kinds of foods can worsen one's condition. He or she should also avoid potatoes, eggplants and tomatoes because these are part of the nightshade family of plant that contains solanine that can provoke the pain. Cutting these kinds of vegetables in people with arthritis have not been proven yet to be effective, but those who followed this kind of diet often show improvements with their condition and find relief from pain.

What are the foods to be added in your diet if you have arthritis? If you already know which kinds of foods you should eliminate in your anti-inflammatory diet, you should now know foods to add to your diet:

1. Healthy fats and Oils: Fish oils are high in Omega-3 fatty acids that are essential to our health. This will help reduce the inflammation and prevent it from coming back. You will also get these fats in some seeds like flaxseed, pumpkin seeds, and sunflower seeds and also in Brazil nuts, almonds, cashew nuts and many more.

2. Fruits and Vegetables: You should be eating more fruits and vegetables if you have arthritis because these have a lot of mineral, vitamins, antioxidants and photochemical that are beneficial for your arthritis and also to other conditions.

3. Protein: Eating more proteins like fishes and other seafoods and poultry meats will also help people with arthritis.

4. Drinks: You should need more liquids to keep your joints lubricated. Drink more water, fruit juices, tea, vegetable juice with low sodium and non-fat milk.

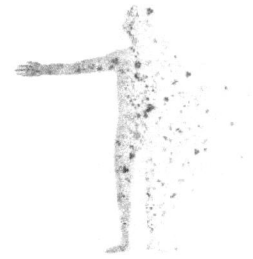

Most people who experience inflammation have heard all about the medications that are available to cure the pain and swelling that can occur during a flare up. But how many know that there are some great anti inflammatory foods that can affect how you feel and reduce the pain associated with inflammation.

Following an anti inflammatory diet will help you beat inflammation naturally.

Inflammation is a swelling that may cause pain, discoloration and even the loss of movement. Usually most people experience severe inflammation when they are the sufferers of arthritis and when they have problems like heart disease and strokes.

Usually your doctor will recommend that you get sleep and exercise in moderation. He may also suggest lowering your weight and taking steroid based drugs or undergoing joint replacement surgery. The medications do work fairly well in reducing the inflammation but often come with some serious side effects, such as ulcers and kidney problems. This may make you wonder if they are worth taking and whether using them is trading one illness for another.

Just like there are some foods that decrease inflammation, there are some that will increase the likelihood that you will get inflammation. These foods are junk foods, fast foods, sugar, and fatty meats. Processed foods that contain Trans and saturated fats also increase the risk of inflammation. Other large contributors of saturated fats are dairy products and eggs. By simply choosing low fat milk, low fat cheese and leaner cuts of meat, you can lower the risks of inflammation, as well as cut down on the chances of chronic disease and obesity. Other foods that increase inflammation include presweetened cereals and soft drinks.

In addition to these, there are foods that are high in sugar and foods that come from the plants labeled as nightshade type. These add to the risk of discomfort associated with inflammation. Eating whole fruits and vegetables will give you the natural healing factors. However, not all vegetables work that way. Potatoes, eggplant and tomatoes can actually make inflammation worse.

So remember the best foods to have are whole fruits, fresh vegetables, lean meats, low fat milk and cheese, as well as fruit and vegetable juices that contain carrots and celery. These types of foods will reduce inflammation and help you get on with your life without pain. Eating right will help you beat inflammation naturally.

A Key to Eating Well

You are what you eat' implies that certain foods can be good or bad for you. They are bad if they are inflammatory foods and good if they are not. If you are a doctor who treats inflammatory conditions, like neck pain or low back pain, wouldn't you want your patients to eat foods that help to reduce inflammation as oppose to consuming inflammatory foods? But how can you tell?

What patients eat can affect their outcome. As a Baltimore chiropractor I have found that review of the literature not only reveals the answer but provides the perfect guide to eating well. So, this article begins with the premise that eating certain foods can actually make things hurt worse-increases inflammation-while eating other foods can actually help lessen pain and promote faster healing. These are known as anti-inflammatory foods and they are closely related to competing omega fatty acids. Swelling, redness, heat and pain occur when tissue become inflamed. It may be overt, like a sprained ankle, or hidden beneath the skin, like in your stomach.

So, what foods should or shouldn't be consumed and why? An example of inflammatory foods are those high in refined or hydrogenated vegetable oils, like potato chips and many baked goods. Refined oils and trans fats are used by manufacturers to extend the shelf life of their products. They are notorious preservatives. On the another hand, olive oil, avocado oil and grape seed oil are natural and are known to be anti-inflammatory. Salmon is very high on the list of ant-inflammatory foods.

The reason has to do with the competing omega fatty acids. "A healthy diet contains a balance of omega-3 and omega-6 fatty acids. Omega-3 fatty acids help reduce inflammation, and some omega-6 fatty acids tend to promote inflammation. The typical American diet tends to contain 14 - 25 times more omega-6 fatty acids than omega-3 fatty acids," according to an excerpt by the University of Maryland Medical System. Now, red meats, such as a good, juicy steak, are high in omega-6 fatty acids. So, does that make it bad? No! It's extremely good for you. A good steak is loaded with essential amino acids and other nutrients. It's just that the key to improving health and reducing inflammation is to balance the amount of omega-6 (e.g., nuts, eggs, poultry, cream, cheese, butter) against the omega-3 (e.g., salmon, tuna, turkey). The saturated fats contained in omega-6 foods compete with the omega-3 foods for vital digestive enzymes, like seagulls fighting over french fries on the boardwalk.

So here's my advice: Limit fatty animal products like red meats and dairy products. Instead, eat more lean cuts of chicken, turkey and fish. Olive oils and avocado can and should replace unhealthy oils from corn, soybeans, safflower, sunflower and other vegetable oils. Sweets should be limited, including all bakery products like cookies, cakes, pies and breads. We all know that our modern diet of processed and fast foods tends to generate inflammation and other evils, like obesity. To counteract bad eating, give close consideration to the competing omega fatty acids.

195

Here's a suggestion: Quinoa and avocado salad (SERVES 4)

INGREDIENTS:

1 cup red quinoa

2 avocados, cut up in

pieces A few dried

tomatoes

2 fresh basil leaves

1 green onion

Dressing:

½ cup olive oil

Juice of 2 lemons

1 garlic clove (minced)

Salt

Cayenne (very small amount)

DIRECTIONS:

Rinse quinoa in cold water and drain well

In saucepan, bring 2 cups water and ½ tsp. salt to boil. Add quinoa. Cover and reduce heat to low. Cook until water is absorbed (about 20 minutes).

In a bowl, mix together the ingredients in cooled quinoa. Toss with dressing.

AVOIDING INFLAMMATORY FOODS

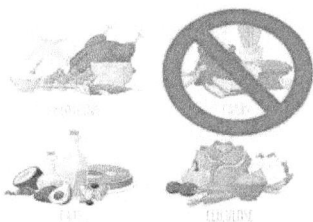

Chronic inflammation continues to threaten the lives of millions worldwide. Today, people are suffering from illnesses such as cardiovascular disease, respiratory disorders, cancers and other inflammatory ailments including familial Mediterranean fever. Developing countries are especially prone to such illnesses and often die from various cancers. Many studies today have shown that lifestyle choices, especially foods we consume everyday, can greatly impact the rate of illnesses.

A well-balanced diet can help fight many of the illnesses people are faced with every day. Some of these foods have anti-inflammatory compounds, which can deter the body from such diseases. As a result, avoiding inflammatory promoting foods and consuming more natural anti-inflammatory foods will greatly reduce the number of illnesses. Here are just a few of the foods that you should avoid which often sets the stage for this inflammatory illnesses.

Alcohol

Found in wines, liquors, and beer, alcohol is often the onset of inflammation in the liver, larynx and esophagus. Chronic inflammation can also develop which promotes tumor growths.

Sugar

Sugar is found in all kinds of candy, desserts, snacks, and beverages. Unfortunately though, excessive amounts of sugar can lead to chronic diseases such as type 2 diabetes, and risk of obesity in addition to inflammatory disorders such as familial Mediterranean fever.

Processed Red Meat

Processed red meat can be found in beef, pork, lamb, salami, and more and should be a red flag. They contain a molecule known as Neu5Gc, which humans do not naturally produce. As a result, ingesting this compound can trigger inflammatory response from the developed anti-Neu5Gc antibodies. These animal products have been known to contribute to colon and rectum cancer in addition to lung and esophagus cancer.

Common Cooking Oils

Cooking oils contain elevated levels of omega-6 fatty acids and low levels of omega-3 fats, not to mention, promotes inflammation and disorders including familial Mediterranean fever. They are used in processed foods and should be avoided at all times.

Artificial Food Additives

Certain food additives are known to trigger inflammation especially in those individuals suffering from conditions like rheumatoid arthritis. These food additives are known as MSG, or monosodium glutamate, and aspartame, which are taste enhancers.

Trans Fats

Trans fats have the tendency of elevated "bad" cholesterol levels while diminishing "good" cholesterol levels, in addition to promoting obesity, insulin resistance and inflammation. They are found in most fast foods, deep fried foods, and commercial baked goods.

Dairy Products

Dairy products are consumed by many people but can not be properly digested. Milk for example, is a common allergen known to induce inflammation and other responses in the intestinal tract. These can all result in constipation, stomach distress, acne, diarrhea, hives, skin rashes, and difficulty breathing.

Refined Grains

Many of the grains consumed today are refined and lack any vitamin B or fiber. They are found in items such as pastries, biscuits, white rice, white bread, white flour, pasta and noodles, and are comparable to refined sugars, however, have an even higher glycemic index, and can trigger degenerative diseases.

Common Inflammatory Arthritis Types

Inflammatory arthritis is arthritis which will inflame the joints. There are many types of this type of arthritis, but to simplify it, I am only going to go over a few types and tell what these types are specifically.

One of the most common inflammatory arthritis types is rheumatoid arthritis. Rheumatoid arthritis can cause a variety of joint pain symptoms as well as other symptoms that make you feel unwell. The symptoms of rheumatoid arthritis are those such as:

1. Intensive joint pains

2. Inflammation of the joints causing swelling

3. Sometimes you may have a rash

4. Fever may be present

Diagnosis of Rheumatoid Arthritis involves something called a SED-RATE blood test. This test will show abnormal results in mostly all people that have rheumatoid arthritis. Another very important test the rheumatologist will certainly do is the blood test which tells the rheumatoid factor in the blood. That factor is always high in the case of people with rheumatoid arthritis.

Upon finding out that Rheumatoid Arthritis is the case, treatments will begin with anti-inflammatory drugs along with a cancer fighting drug called Methotrexate, which my mom has taken for years for rheumatoid arthritis. Methotrexate does wonders for pain reduction of rheumatoid arthritis and helps the person be able to live a happier pain-free life.

Doctors might also use steroid pills or injections to reduce the pain from Rheumatoid Arthritis.

Another inflammatory arthritis type is actually Systemic Lupus. Systemic Lupus is very debilitating over time to the person who has it. The disease brings on symptoms such as:

1. Joint pains, inflammation, and a lot of swelling in the extremo.oInflammatory arthritis is arthritis which will inflame the joints. There are many types of this type of arthritis, but to simplify it, I am only going to go over a few types and tell what these types are specifically.

First, you must understand that any type of inflammatory arthritis is an autoimmune disorder. Autoimmune diseases are those which causes the immune system to launch an attack on its own antibodies, causing various types of medical problems. Inflammatory arthritis is arthritis which will inflame the joints. There are many types of this type of arthritis, but to simplify it, I am only going to go over a few types and tell what these types are specifically.

2. There is definitely skin rashes in many places. 3. Headaches 4. Fevers occur 5. Infections, colds, and flu

Systemic Lupus can be very mild, or very severe. Instead of your immune system creating healthy antibodies, in Systemic Lupus, your immune system prefers to create antibodies that attack major organs.

Treatment for Systemic Lupus involves treating the symptoms that radiate from the disease since there is no cure at this time. Drugs that have an anti-inflammatory effect may help, and a diet that contains foods with properties which help bone and joint pains may ease some of the joint discomfort.

Skin medications and creams may help the various skin type of problems with lupus as well as staying out of the bright sunlight.

Another commonly heard about inflammatory arthritis type is Reiter's Syndrome. Reiter's Syndrome is just as bad as Systemic Lupus in that it causes a lot of joint pain and inflammation, and is very life-limiting as far as being free from pain. This condition is one of those joint diseases that progresses step-by-step, going so far as to affect the eyes conjunctiva, tendons that are latched on to the joints, and the whole body's bone structures, (meaning the skeleton). Interestingly enough, this inflammatory arthritis type comes from sexually transmitted diseases. Venereal diseases carry many types of bacteria strains that cause this dreadful disease.

Symptoms of Reiter's Syndrome are:

1. Genitalia pain since it is coming from bacterias there

2. Multiple joint pains all over the body such as elbows, knees, foot joints, and every possible joint thought of.

3. It is common to have many sores and many rashes

People with Reiter's Syndrome are helped up to a point with anti-inflammatory medications, and possibly Methotrexate, heat therapies for all of the joint pains, and nutritional changes may help.

If the underlying venereal disease is cured or controlled, a lot of the pain from Reiter's Syndrome will clear up since this is the main cause to begin with. To avoid Reiter's Syndrome to begin with, be aware of venereal disease with your sexual partner.

Ankylosing Spondylitis is an inflammatory type of arthritis caused by many years of doing athletics. After a certain number of years as an athlete, bones and ligaments get torn. If this sports related injury is not treated on an ongoing basis, then bone problems will continue progressing until Ankylosing Spondylitis developments within the connective tissues.

This bone issue begins within the sacroiliac joints. This is where both the pelvis and lower spine join together. The symptoms are:

1. Intense back pains

2. Tiredness

3. Trouble with relaxation and breathing very deeply

4. Painful, swollen, red eyes

Treatment for Ankylosing Spondylitis involves getting the immune system back up to where it should be, and the use of steroids and doing blood testing trying to find the reasons for antibodies not functioning properly in the first place. Some of the causes can be due to allergies in foods, and other infectious cycles taking place within the body itself.

FISH OIL'S ROLE IN REDUCING SYMPTOMS OF INFLAMMATORY BOWEL DISEASE (IBD) AND CROHN'S DISEASE

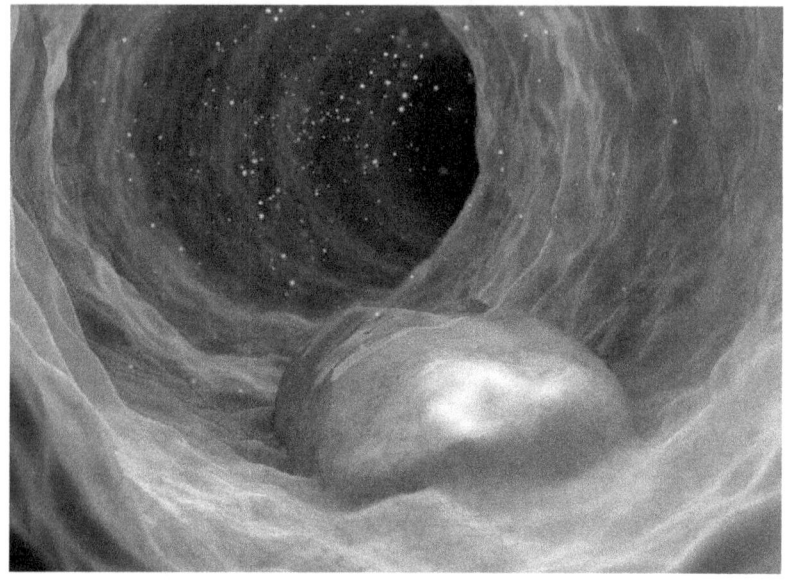

With each passing medical and scientific study the benefits of fish oil and fish oil supplements, are finding their way into the spotlight. Many studies have shown a correlation between reducing the possibility of heart failure, heart attack and different vascular diseases, but it has only been recently that a connection between Omega-3 fatty acids and helpful benefits for patients suffering from Irritable Bowl Diseases (IBDs) such as ulcerative colitis and Chrohn's disease.

Many of these studies are double-blind studies that are further validated with cultural studies of Inuit and Eskimo populations that have a diet high in fish that contains Omega-3 fatty acids and a very low occurrence of ulcerative colitis and Chrohn's disease.

As the evidence mounts, further studies will be needed to pinpoint with any accuracy how much the dietary intake of Omega-3 fatty acids can help in patients suffering from these gastrointestinal diseases, but on the surface the smaller studies that have been done are very promising.

Ulcerative Colitis and Chrohn's Disease Overview

Ulcerative Colitis and Crohn's disease are two types of inflammatory bowel diseases. These diseases are believed to be caused by several factors. First, genetic and non-genetic causes are believed to be the culprit in many cases. The other possible cause is environmental factors such as infections that cause an immune reaction in the gastrointestinal area. The body then generates a large amount of white blood cells in the intestinal lining. These white blood cells release chemicals in the process of fighting the infection that inflame the intestinal tissue. It should be noted, though, that the exact causes of IBDs, such as ulcerative colitis and Crohn's disease, are currently unknown.

In general, an ulcerative colitis attack or Crohn's disease attack will consist of severe intestinal inflammation, which can cause bloody diarrhea, stomach cramps, fever, loss of appetite, weight loss, anemia, bleeding from the ulcers, rupture of the bowel, obstructions and strictures, fistulae, toxic megacolon and malignant cancer. In the last instance, the risk of colon cancer in patients that have had ulcerative colitis or Crohn's disease rises significantly. Generally, after an attack, the disease will go into a remission stage that can last weeks or even years. If you are suffering from these symptoms you should see your physician immediately for a proper diagnosis.

Until recently, the treatment for ulcerative colitis and Crohn's disease was, first and foremost, a healthy diet. If symptoms require it, physicians will ask their patients to limit their intake of dairy and fiber. While it is true that diet has relatively little to no influence on the actual inflammation process within ulcerative colitis, it could have influence on the different symptoms associated with it. On the other hand, diet does have an impact on the inflammatory activity in Crohn's disease and one of the main ways of treating these symptoms is a diet that consists of predigested food. It should also be noted that in both diseases, stress has been shown to be a factor in causing flare-ups. Because of this, physicians will also emphasize the importance of stress management.

Secondarily, medical treatment for these two diseases involves suppression of the high level of inflammatory response mechanisms of the immune system within the intestinal tract. By suppressing this response, the intestinal tissue can heal and the symptoms of abdominal pain and diarrhea can be relieved. After the symptoms have been controlled, further medicinal treatment helps to decrease flare-ups and lengthen or maintain remission periods.

Conventional methods of medicating these two diseases involve a stepped approach. Initially, the least harmful of medications are given in as low a dosage as possible and are taken for a short time period. If these medications provide little or no relief, the dosages are either increased or the medications are changed.

The lowest levels of medications, or Step I, are aminosalicylates and antibiotics. Corticosteroids make up the set of Step II drugs. Step III drugs involve the use of immune modifying medications or a drug called Infliximab for patients suffering from Crohn's disease. These medications are not used, however, during acute flare-ups due to the length of time that a flare-up can last. Only after Step III medications fail completely are Step IV drugs introduced because at this time, they are experimental.

A final alternative in treating ulcerative colitis is surgery. Because ulcerative colitis is limited to the colon, surgery can completely cure it. Crohn's disease, unfortunately, is not restricted to the colon and can exist anywhere in the digestive tract. Because of this, surgery will often complicate matters more.

Limitations of Medical Treatment

Nearly one-quarter of all patients diagnosed with some form of IBD, either Crohn's disease or ulcerative colitis, will not respond to medical treatment. In about three-quarters of cases of Crohn's disease, surgery (even though it is not curative) will be required. Regardless of current medical treatment, a person suffering from ulcerative colitis will have a 50% chance of having remission end within a two-year period after the last flare-up. Even if the initial diagnosis of ulcerative colitis is limited to the rectum there is a 50% probability of the disease becoming more extensive over a twenty-five year period. If a patient has ulcerative colitis that involves the entire colon, that patient stands a 60% chance of requiring a colectomy and most patients will require surgical intervention within the first year after diagnosis of the disease.

It's obvious that Intestinal Bowel Disease can be debilitating. Continued treatments with progressively harsher medications and surgeries that may help in some cases but not others become the norm for these patients. Further, the complications like strictures and fistulas associated with IBDs, can ultimately lead to colon cancer. Many times, these complications create a feeling of hopelessness among those who suffer from ulcerative colitis or Crohn's disease.

There is hope, though. New studies are presenting strong evidence for the use of Omega-3 fatty acids (fish oil and fish oil supplements) in the prevention and treatment of IBDs. These studies are shedding new light on the multi-faceted health benefits of Omega-3 fatty acids and ultimately may present new methods for the treatment of this painful diseases.

The Case for Omega-3 Fatty Acids

Traditionally, the Inuit populations of Alaska have existed on diets high in fatty fish, specifically, types of fish that are high in Omega-3 fatty acids. Past studies of these cultures have shown that the large majority of these groups do not suffer from heart

207

problems, heart disease or other forms of vascular disease. Less known, however, was the fact that the majority of people within these cultures also do not suffer from any form of Inflammatory Bowel Disease. This has led some scientists to postulate that there is a strong connection between the dietary intake of fish oil or fish oil supplements and the prevention of IBDs.

Take, for instance, one example of a symptom of both Crohn's disease and ulcerative colitis: inflammation. Fish oils high in Omega-3 fatty acids have anti-inflammatory properties, which can help reduce its occurrence in patients suffering from IBDs. The reason for this is that when Omega-3 fatty acids are introduced into the body it suppresses the production of leukotriene B4. Omega-3s have also been shown to inhibit interleukin 1Beta. Both leukotriene B4 and interleukin 1Beta are major players in the inflammation of mucosa lining the gastrointestinal tracts.

With regular dietary intake of fish oil supplements high in DHA (docosahexaenoic acid) and EPA (eicosapentaenoic acid), inflammation can be reduced by up to 50% in the intestinal tissues of patients who suffer from ulcerative colitis. Fish oils that have anti-inflammatory properties are only effective in reducing inflammation, but not preventing it. Results in patients with Crohn's disease haven't been quite as promising, but this area of research is still in its infancy.

Recent studies show tremendous promise in fish oil's effectiveness in preventing and reducing the effects of IBDs. These studies show that there is an increase in the manufacture of less powerful prostaglandins at the sacrifice of the more potent ones. Patients with active ulcerative colitis who were given fish oil supplements have also shown significant improvement versus patients who were given placebos. Further study with larger control groups is needed, though, in order for more accurate data to be gathered.

As further evidence of the link between Omega-3s and relief from the symptoms and inflammation of IBDs, a 12-week study involving patients who knew they were taking fish oil supplements showed a significant decline in the disease. This study was further bolstered by the results from samples of the intestinal mucosa that were found to have increased amounts of eicosapentaenoic acid. These results increase when the supplement given to the patients is encased with an enteric coating, which allows the fish oil to be released lower into the intestinal tract. This further alleviates side effects such as fishy breath, burping and flatulence related to taking fish oil supplements. Because of the fewer side effects associated with these supplements, treatment over the long-term is more tolerable.

A Worldwide Phenomenon

With more notice being taken of the effects of Omega-3 fatty acids on the health of people who take them on a consistent basis, the worldwide scientific community has opened up more to the idea of this supplement being used for effective treatment of IBDs. For instance, in Italy, a study was conducted using enteric-coated fish oil supplements and a notable reduction in the rate of relapse in Crohn's disease remission was noted. The patients involved in this study showed evidence of inflammation at the beginning of the study and were suffering from the symptoms related to Crohn's. In this study, patients suffering from the disease received either three fish oil capsules three times per day or a placebo three times per day. Those patients receiving fish oil supplements showed a significant reduction in the inflammation.

Among 39 patients in the placebo group, almost 70% of the patients who were in remission, relapsed. Out of the 39 patients supplementing their diet with fish oil capsules, only 28% relapsed. Further, after a year, nearly 60% of the 39 patients being given fish oil supplements were still in remission while only 25% of the patients given the placebo were in remission.

Given the small size of the study group it is only possible to speculate on the efficacy of treatment for Crohn's disease patients, however, the results of this study are promising. If scientists are given the opportunity to produce a study with a much larger group of patients, better and more accurate data could be gathered which could lead to even more positive results. More research would also allow scientists and doctors to understand the ways in which the EPA works to help increase time of remission.

There is strong speculation that patients suffering from IBDs lack a particular enzyme found in Omega-3 pathways and that when this enzyme is present, remission and even prevention of IBDs is possible. In a sense, adding an Omega-3 supplement to the diet of a patient suffering from Crohn's disease or ulcerative colitis appears to be a type of enzyme replacement therapy.

In Japan, medical researchers at Shiga University of Medical Science conducted a study in which the diet of Crohn's disease patients was altered to include a meal of rice, cooked fish and soup. Prior to the establishment of this diet, the occurrence of relapse within one year was 90%. After implementation of the diet the occurrence of relapse dropped to 40% within one year. Results like this are encouraging other countries to do similar studies.

In the United States, research conducted at Boston University Medical Center shows that patients with chronic IBD have unusual fatty acid profiles that were generally lower than control subjects who did not suffer from any type of chronic intestinal disorder. Because of this lack of fatty acids it is believed that these patients are more prone to these problems. The study also suggests that the addition of Omega-3 fatty acids via a diet that adds fish oil or fish oil supplements can help reduce and correct this shortage.

Another study in San Francisco that involved patients with ulcerative colitis showed that there is an increase in leukotriene B4 in the colonic lining. The hypothesis in this study is that an increase in fish oil supplements in patients suffering from ulcerative colitis could inhibit the synthesis of the leukotrienes. If this is possible, fish oil supplements would be responsible for a reduction or elimination of the symptoms associated with inflammation of the bowels in this disease.

The final results of the study show that the hypothesis was accurate. Patients in the study were randomized and placed into two different groups. The study group received regular daily doses of fish oil containing 2.7 grams of eicosapentaenoic acid and 1.8

grams of docosahexaenoic acid. The second set of patients were placed into a control group and given placebo capsules filled with olive oil. Over a three-month period, patients receiving the fish oil supplements showed marked improvement in the severity of the symptoms of the disease. In fact, 72% of the study group taking the supplements was able to reduce or completely terminate their anti-inflammation and steroid medication schedules.

A similar study done at Mount Sinai School of Medicine shows that the regular use of fish oil supplements in patients suffering from ulcerative colitis diminishes the severity of the disease. Fully 70% of the patients involved in the study showed moderate to significant improvement and 80% of the patients in the study were able to reduce their intake of prednisone, an anti-inflammatory used to help alleviate symptoms of the disease, by up to 66%.

Taking the Next Steps

Studies are showing positive results and it's obvious that the Omega-3 fatty acids inherent to fish oil supplements are beneficial to our intestinal health. The obvious thing to do is find out what types of fish oil supplements are the best. Personal research will aid you in finding the correct supplements and additionally if you suffer from Crohn's disease or ulcerative colitis, you should consult with your physician about the benefits of adding a fish oil supplement to your diet and what dosage you should take. There is, however, some basic information about fish oil supplements that you need to know.

First of all, not all fish oil supplements are created equal. Cod liver oil is, by far, the most inexpensive form of fish oil that contains Omega-3 fatty acids. However, it does not contain the highest amounts and in most cases it cannot be taken in high doses because of impurities such as mercury that are left in it. It also has an extremely powerful taste that most have trouble tolerating.

A much better choice for supplementing your diet with fish oil is a health food grade supplement. These supplements have been purified using a process called molecular distillation. This process eliminates nearly all of the impurities and is very safe when taken in the doses necessary to help alleviate the symptoms associated with IBDs.

The purest form of fish oil supplements is pharmaceutical grade. These supplements have also been processed using molecular distillation, however, at a much higher level. The process used in filtering out the impurities gets rid of all of them down to the particulate level. These supplements, of course, are also the most expensive, but will have the greatest impact on your ulcerative colitis or Crohn's disease.

The benefits of Omega-3 fatty acids are proving to be phenomenal and it is anyone's guess as to the limits of what these supplements can do for our health. With few side effects that are relatively minor, fish oil supplements are a good choice to help you improve your overall health. The fact that they can be used to inhibit the relapse of the symptoms of Crohn's disease and ulcerative colitis is even more exciting. Omega-3 fatty acids are carving out a healthy niche in the diets of individuals worldwide and everyone is all the better for it.

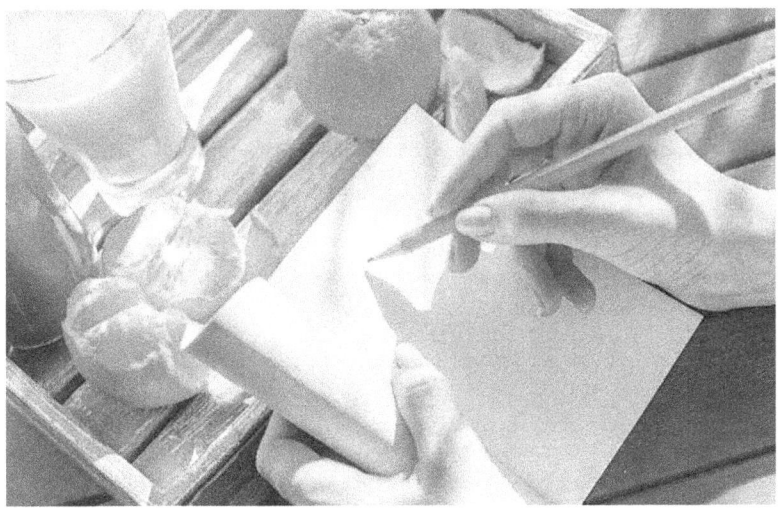

Many diseases such as cancer, cardiovascular disease and autoimmune diseases such as rheumatoid arthritis and celiac disease are linked to chronic inflammation in the body. Luckily, there are many ways to fight inflammation through healthy dietary and lifestyle changes. First and foremost, any dietary modification should begin with a healthy foundation. This includes a balance of lean proteins and healthy fats with a wide variety of colorful fruits, vegetables, grains, and legumes. Variety is the key as focusing on one food, color or nutrient will prevent one from reaping the benefits of all of the others.

There are also many well-known anti-inflammatory foods and nutrients. One of the most researched is omega-3 fatty acids, which are polyunsaturated fats found in foods such as fatty fish like wild salmon, tuna and mackerel, walnuts, chia, flax, and canola oil. A diet rich in antioxidants that includes foods rich in Vitamin C, Vitamin E, and beta-carotene is also known to resist and repair the damage that is induced by inflammation. In addition, phytochemicals in plant foods can also protect against inflammation. Some examples include lycopene, ursolic acid, and lutein. Herbs and spices including turmeric and ginger are also known to have anti-inflammatory properties.

Here are some easy ways to implement an anti-inflammatory diet along with a sample meal plan to help get you started:

Consume a Mediterranean style diet rich in healthy fats such as fish, olive oil, and canola oil; colorful fruits and vegetables; whole grains such as whole wheat pasta and brown rice; and small amounts of lean meats such as skinless poultry breast.

Consume more omega-3 fatty acids from sources such as wild salmon, tuna and mackerel, walnuts, flax, canola oil, omega-fortified eggs. Fish oil supplements that contain both EPA and DHA can be taken under the guidance of your physician.

Consume monounsaturated fat from sources such as avocado, olive oil, and almonds.

Consume more antioxidant-rich fruits and vegetables full of vitamins C, E, and Beta-carotene. Vitamin C can be found in foods such as citrus fruits (oranges, grapefruit), green and red pepper, kiwi, tomatoes, broccoli, and fortified foods. Vitamin E can be found in foods such as wheat germ, vegetable oils, nuts and seeds. Beta-carotene can be found in foods such as carrots, sweet potato, cantaloupe, red pepper, mango, and broccoli

Consume more colorful fruits and vegetables full of phytochemicals such as lycopene, lutein, and ursolic acid. Lycopene can be found in tomatoes, watermelon and red grapefruit. Lutein can be found in dark green leafy vegetables like spinach. Ursolic acid can be found in cranberries, prunes, and apples

Cook with flavorful herbs and spices such as ginger and turmeric. Ginger can be added to soups, stir fry, and homemade tea. Turmeric is used to make curry, casseroles, soups, and stews.

Avoid processed foods, convenience foods, and fast foods which do not contain the healthful properties of an anti-inflammatory diet and contain excessive sodium, preservatives, and saturated fats.

Anti Inflammatory Meal Plan

Breakfast: Add ½ cup berries and ¼ cup shaved almonds to hot or cold cereal

Snack on fruit with low fat or non-fat yogurt or cottage cheese

Lunch: Have a salad with Romaine lettuce, and at least 3 other vegetables that you enjoy (example: carrots, tomatoes, red onions, and cucumber) topped with beans or unsalted plain nuts and olive oil as a dressing

Snack on carrots dipped in hummus

Dinner: Have a stir fry using canola oil including chicken, ground or grated ginger, and red, yellow, and green peppers over brown rice

Snack on a homemade fruit smoothie made with banana, strawberries mixed with skim milk or non-fat yogurt and a tablespoon of ground flax seed.

ANTI-INFLAMMATION DIET FOR DUMMIES CHEAT SHEET

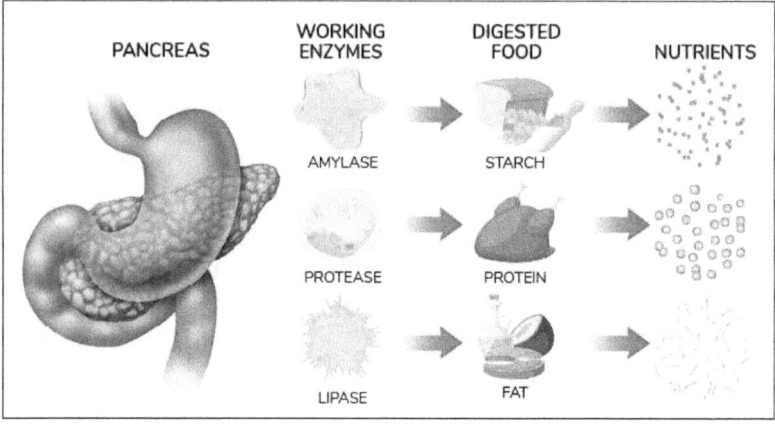

Choosing an anti-inflammation diet is one way to control inflammation in your body. For anyone living with chronic inflammation, finding a way to decrease symptoms and, if possible, erase the inflammation altogether, is a blessing. In many cases, living with inflammation doesn't have to be permanent you can treat, prevent, and sometimes even eradicate those inflammatory issues by knowing which foods are triggers for you, which foods are bad for everyone, and how to change your diet accordingly.

Linking Inflammation to Chronic Diseases

Inflammation contributes to the development and symptoms of chronic illnesses, and understanding that link is the first step in knowing how to change your diet in order to combat inflammation and take better care of yourself. Here are some illnesses linked to inflammation:

216

Heart disease: Clinical research has linked heart disease from coronary artery disease to congestive heart failure to inflammation. Physicians and researchers provide evidence that the fatty deposits the body uses to repair damage to the arteries are just the start.

Cancer: Foods and proteins, such as fruits and green vegetables, can help you significantly reduce your risks of cancer. Chronic inflammation has been shown to contribute to the growth of tumor cells and other cancer cells.

Arthritis and joint pain: Arthritis has always been linked to inflammation, but it hasn't always been evident that a change in diet could help alleviate the pain and possibly even postpone the onset. Now, however, medical and nutrition professionals see the benefits that natural, vitamin-rich foods can have in relieving the pain of arthritis and possibly even diminishing the inflammation.

Weight gain: It's no secret that food is linked to obesity, but certain foods have a tendency to pile on the pounds more than others. Refined flours and sugars, for example, don't get digested properly and turn to fat much sooner than other, unprocessed foods. Obesity increases inflammation throughout the body by piling pressure on the joints and aiding arthritis, for instance.

Choosing Good Fats for an Anti-Inflammation Diet

Consuming fat in an anti-inflammatory diet isn't forbidden — but the key is knowing which fats are good, which are bad, and which aren't too awful in moderation. "Fat" has become a dirty word in the dietary world, but some fats are not only good for you but necessary for a healthy lifestyle:

Good fats: Polyunsaturated and monounsaturated fats are essential to keeping the good fat in your body in check. Good sources of these fats include olive oil, nuts (almonds, pecans, peanuts, and walnuts, for example), oatmeal, sesame oil and seeds, and soybeans, as well as the omega-3 fatty acids found in salmon, herring, trout, and sardines. The total fat intake for a day should equal between 20 and 35 percent of total calories for the day, and just 10 percent of those calories should be made up of the "bad" fats.

Not-so-good fats: Some foods with saturated fats are okay in moderation, as long as your "moderation" doesn't mean daily. Splurge every now and then, but remember that each splurge takes away from the good you're doing for your body. Sources of saturated fats include fatty meats, butter, cheese, ice cream, and palm oil. Not all saturated fats are bad: Coconut and coconut oil, while considered saturated fats, are actually healthy and beneficial to an anti-inflammatory diet.

Awful fats: Avoid trans fats at all costs. Trans fats are the bad fats found in cakes, pastries, margarine, and shortening, among other foods. One quick and easy way to identify trans fats is to consider the form: Is the fat a solid that can melt and then solidify again? If so, chances are it's a trans fat. Reading the labels on foods is another way to identify trans fats: Hydrogenated or partially hydrogenated fats are trans fats, too.

Making Anti-Inflammatory Food Choices

After you discover the link between inflammation and chronic illness — and the important role food has in fighting them both — you need an idea of what foods will help you treat and even prevent inflammation. Here are some ideas to guide your food choices for different meals:

Breakfasts: Turn to natural ingredients in homemade smoothies, such as berries, honey, and Greek or non-dairy yogurt. Some egg dishes, particularly those made with organic eggs, can help lower inflammation as well. Want toast? Try something gluten- and wheat-free, like rice breads.

Snacks and appetizers: The easiest natural snack is a handful of fruit or fresh veggies. Grab a good crispy apple or a handful of snow peas and you've done your body proud. Want to make it a little snappier? Throw together an avocado dip, stuff an oversized portobello mushroom with kale and other heart-healthy ingredients, or grab a handful of dates. Fruits and nuts are great on-the-go snacks and are filled with vitamins and nutrients, as well as the benefits of omega-3 fatty acids found in most nuts.

Soups and salads: Sometimes there's nothing better than a good cup of soup or a nice salad, but it's easy to get fooled by those that may not be as healthy as they appear. Good soups for fighting inflammation include vegetable soup with a butternut squash base or miso soup with gluten-free noodles. Many people have inflammatory reactions to tomatoes and other nightshade fruits and vegetables, so it's a good idea to stay away from tomato-based soups with potatoes and bell peppers. For salads, steer toward the darker greens and fresh organic toppers, dressed with just a sprinkling of vinegar or olive oil.

Main dishes: Some good anti-inflammatory options for main dishes include most kinds of fish, which is full of omega-3 fatty acids. If you're looking for a bit of protein in your main dish, turn to chicken or even tofu. Try to avoid red meat if possible, but use grass-fed meat if you must go that route.

Desserts: Think "desserts" and the word "sweet" is likely the first to pop into mind — and just because you're trying to fight inflammation doesn't mean you have to fight your sweet tooth, too. Try some chopped fruit and melted dark chocolate to get the vitamins in the fruit and the rich antioxidants in dark chocolate. Need something creamy? Try adding some vanilla extract or honey to a Greek or non-dairy yogurt or, if dairy isn't a problem for you, add it to a little bit of light ricotta cheese.

Changing Your Cooking Methods to Reduce Inflammation

An anti-inflammatory diet begins with choosing the right foods, but it continues with using anti-inflammatory cooking methods to prepare those foods. You can undo a lot of the good in your healthy foods by cooking them the wrong way. Here are some tips on getting the most out of your cooking methods:

Baking: Put your food in the center of a glass or ceramic baking dish, leaving room around the sides to let hot air circulate. Setting veggies on the bottom of a dish, under meat or fish, adds moisture and enhances flavor. Cover the dish to let the food cook with steam while retaining its natural juices.

Steaming: Use a vegetable steamer, rice cooker, or bamboo steamer or create your own steamer with a covered pot and slotted insert to gently cook a variety of foods. Take care, not to overcook vegetables, fish, or seafood. Marinate foods with herbs such as rosemary and sage before steaming, and add spices such as ginger and turmeric to foods while steaming to infuse the flavor into the food.

Poaching: This gentle cooking method requires no additional fats, such as oil. Bring poaching liquid (water or stock, usually) to a boil and add your meat, seafood, or veggies; reduce the heat and simmer until done for a low-fat, flavorful result. Save the poaching liquid from meat or fish and use it as the base of a soup.

Stir-frying: This method allows you to cook with a small amount of oil (or none at all) at high temperatures for a very short amount of time so that the food absorbs very little oil. Vegetables in particular retain their beneficial nutrients.

Grilling and broiling: Reserve grilling for fish and veggies, which don't need much cooking time. Grilling and broiling meats involves excessive temperatures that cause the fats and proteins in meat and protein turn into heterocyclic amines (HAs), which may raise the risk of certain cancers.

Microwaving: As for giving your food a quick zap in the microwave, that convenience appliance destroys the nutrients in food because of the high heat, so you should avoid this cooking method.

RULES FOR OPTIMAL HEALTH OF ANTI-INFLAMMATORY DIETS

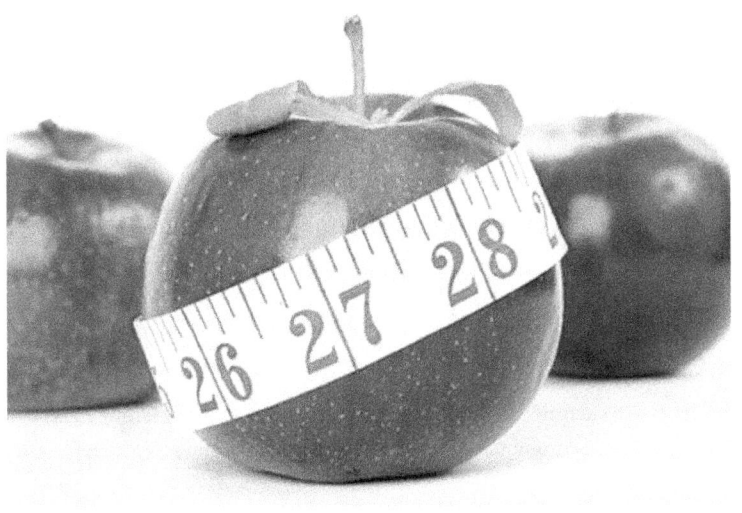

If you want to eat for long-term health, lowering inflammation is crucial. Inflammation in the body causes or contributes to many debilitating, chronic illnesses—including osteoarthritis, rheumatoid arthritis, heart disease, Alzheimer's disease, Parkinson's disease, and even cancer.

Recent research finds that eating this way not only helps protect against certain diseases, but it also slows the aging process by stabilizing blood sugar and increasing metabolism.

Plus, although the goal is to optimize health, many people find they also lose weight by following an anti-inflammatory eating pattern. If you're interested in figuring out what overall diet (Mediterranean, Paleo, etc) is best for inflammation, this is a great article to check out. In general, though, I recommend everyone follow these 11 principles:

1. Consume at least 25 grams of fiber every day.

A fiber-rich diet helps reduce inflammation by supplying naturally occurring anti-inflammatory phytonutrients found in fruits, vegetables, and other whole foods.

To get your fill of fiber, seek out whole grains, fruits, and vegetables. The best sources include whole grains such as barley and oatmeal; vegetables like okra, eggplant, and onions; and a variety of fruits like bananas (3 grams of fiber per banana) and blueberries (3.5 grams of fiber per cup).

2. Eat a minimum of nine servings of fruits and vegetables every day.

One "serving" is half a cup of a cooked fruit or vegetable, or one cup of a raw leafy vegetable.

For an extra punch, add anti-inflammatory herbs and spices — such as turmeric and ginger — to your cooked fruits and vegetables to increase their antioxidant capacity.

3. Eat four servings of both alliums and crucifers every week.

Alliums include garlic, scallions, onions, and leek, while crucifers refer to vegetables such as broccoli, cabbage, cauliflower, mustard greens, and Brussels sprouts.

Because of their powerful antioxidant properties, consuming a weekly average of four servings of each can help lower your risk of cancer.

4. Limit saturated fat to 10 percent of your daily calories.

By keeping saturated fat low (that's about 20 grams per 2,000 calories), you'll help reduce the risk of heart disease.

You should also limit red meat to once per week and marinate it with herbs, spices, and tart, unsweetened fruit juices to reduce the toxic compounds formed during cooking.

5. Consume foods rich in omega-3 fatty acids.

Research shows that omega-3 fatty acids reduce inflammation and may help lower risk of chronic diseases such as heart disease, cancer, and arthritis — conditions that often have a high inflammatory process at their root.

Aim to eat lots of foods high in omega-3 fatty acids like flax meal, walnuts, and beans such as navy, kidney and soy. I also recommend taking a good-quality omega-3 supplement.

And of course, consume cold-water fish such as salmon, oysters, herring, mackerel, trout, sardines, and anchovies. Speaking of which:

6. Eat fish at least three times a week.

Choose both low-fat fish such as sole and flounder, and cold-water fish that contain healthy fats, like the ones mentioned above.

7. Use oils that contain healthy fats.

The body requires fat, but choose the fats that provide you with benefits.

Virgin and extra-virgin olive oil (organic if possible like this one) and expeller-pressed canola are the best bets for anti-inflammatory benefits. Other options include high-oleic, expeller-pressed versions of sunflower and safflower oil.

8. Eat healthy snacks twice a day.

If you're a snacker, aim for fruit, plain or unsweetened Greek-style yogurt (it contains more protein per serving), celery sticks, carrots, or nuts like pistachios, almonds, and walnuts.

9. Avoid processed foods and refined sugars.

This includes any food that contains high-fructose corn syrup or is high in sodium, which contribute to inflammation throughout the body.

Avoid refined sugars whenever possible and artificial sweeteners altogether. The dangers of excess fructose have been widely cited and include increased insulin resistance (which can lead to type-2 diabetes), raised uric acid levels, raised blood pressure, increased risk of fatty liver disease, and more.

10. Cut out trans fats.

In 2006, the FDA required food manufacturers to identify trans fats on nutrition labels, and for good reason — studies show that people who eat foods high in trans fats have higher levels of C-reactive protein, a biomarker for inflammation in the body.

A good rule of thumb is to always read labels and steer clear of products that contain the words "hydrogenated" or "partially hydrogenated oils." Vegetable shortenings, select margarines, crackers, and cookies are just a few examples of foods that might contain trans fats.

11. Sweeten meals with phytonutrient-rich fruits, and flavor foods with spices.

Most fruits and vegetables are loaded with important phytonutrients. In order to naturally sweeten your meals, try adding apples, apricots, berries, and even carrots.

And for flavoring savory meals, go for spices that are known for their anti-inflammatory properties, including cloves, cinnamon, turmeric, rosemary, ginger, sage, and thyme.

MAINSTREAM NUTRITION MYTHS

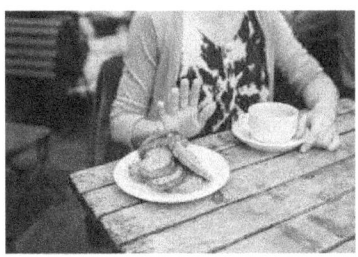

Despite clear advancements in nutrition science, the old myths don't seem to be going anywhere.

Here are 20 mainstream nutrition myths that have been debunked by scientific research.

Myth 1: The Healthiest Diet Is a Low-Fat, High-Carb Diet With Lots of Grains

Several decades ago, the entire population was advised to eat a low-fat, high-carb diet

At the time, not a single study had demonstrated that this diet could actually prevent disease.

Since then, many high quality studies have been done, including the Women's Health Initiative, which is the largest nutrition study in history.

The results were clear... this diet does not cause weight loss, prevent cancer OR reduce the risk of heart disease

Numerous studies have been done on the low-fat, high-carb diet. It has virtually no effect on body weight or disease risk over the long term.

Myth 2: Salt Should Be Restricted in Order to Lower Blood Pressure and Reduce Heart Attacks and Strokes

The salt myth is still alive and kicking, even though there has never been any good scientific support for it.

Although lowering salt can reduce blood pressure by 1-5 mm/Hg on average, it doesn't have any effect on heart attacks, strokes or death.

Of course, if you have a medical condition like salt-sensitive hypertension then you may be an exception.

But the public health advice that everyone should lower their salt intake (and have to eat boring, tasteless food) is not based on evidence.

Despite modestly lowering blood pressure, reducing salt/sodium does not reduce the risk of heart attacks, strokes or death.

Myth 3: It Is Best to Eat Many, Small Meals Throughout the Day to "Stoke the Metabolic Flame"

It is often claimed that people should eat many, small meals throughout the day to keep the metabolism high.

But the studies clearly disagree with this. Eating 2-3 meals per day has the exact same effect on total calories burned as eating 5-6 (or more) smaller meals

Eating frequently may have benefits for some people (like preventing excessive hunger), but it is incorrect that this affects the amount of calories we burn.

There are even studies showing that eating too often can be harmful... a new study came out recently showing that more frequent meals dramatically increased liver and abdominal fat on a high calorie diet.

It is not true that eating many, smaller meals leads to an increase in the amount of calories burned throughout the day. Frequent meals may even increase the accumulation of unhealthy belly and liver fat.

Myth 4: Egg Yolks Should Be Avoided Because They Are High in Cholesterol, Which Drives Heart Disease

We've been advised to cut back on whole eggs because the yolks are high in cholesterol.

However, cholesterol in the diet has remarkably little effect on cholesterol in the blood, at least for the majority of people.

Studies have shown that eggs raise the "good" choleserol and don't raise risk of heart disease

One review of 17 studies with a total of 263,938 participants showed that eating eggs had no effect on the risk of heart disease or stroke in non-diabetic individuals

However... keep in mind that some studies have found an increased heart attack risk in diabetics who eat eggs.

Whole eggs really are among the most nutritious foods on the planet and almost all the nutrients are found in the yolks.

Telling people to throw the yolks away may just be the most ridiculous advice in the history of nutrition.

Despite eggs being high in cholesterol, they do not raise blood cholesterol or increase heart disease risk for the majority of people.

Myth 5: Whole Wheat Is a Health Food and an Essential Part of a "Balanced" Diet"

Wheat has been a part of the diet for a very long time, but it changed due to genetic tampering in the 1960s.

The "new" wheat is significantly less nutritious than the older varieties

Preliminary studies have shown that, compared to older wheat, modern wheat may increase cholesterol levels and inflammatory markers.

It also causes symptoms like pain, bloating, tiredness and reduced quality of life in patients with irritable bowel syndrome.

Whereas some of the older varieties like Einkorn and Kamut may be relatively healthy, modern wheat is not.

Also, let's not forget that the "whole grain" label is a joke... these grains have usually been pulverized into very fine flour, so they have similar metabolic effects as refined grains.

The wheat most people are eating today is unhealthy. It is less nutritious and may increase cholesterol levels and inflammatory markers.

Myth 6: Saturated Fat Raises LDL Cholesterol in the Blood, Increasing Risk of Heart Attacks

For decades, we've been told that saturated fat raises cholesterol and causes heart disease.

In fact, this belief is the cornerstone of modern dietary guidelines.

However... several massive review studies have recently shown that saturated fat is NOT linked to an increased risk of death from heart disease or stroke

The truth is that saturated fats raise HDL (the "good") cholesterol and change the LDL particles from small to Large LDL, which is linked to reduced risk

For most people, eating reasonable amounts of saturated fat is perfectly safe and downright healthy.

Several recent studies have shown that saturated fat consumption does not increase the risk of death from heart disease or stroke.

Myth 7: Coffee Is Unhealthy and Should Be Avoided

Coffee has long been considered unhealthy, mainly because of the caffeine. However, most of the studies actually show that coffee has powerful health benefits.

This may be due to the fact that coffee is the biggest source of antioxidants in the Western diet, outranking both fruits and vegetables.

Coffee drinkers have a much lower risk of depression, type 2 diabetes, Alzheimer's, Parkinson's... and some studies even show that they live longer than people who don't drink coffee.

Despite being perceived as unhealthy, coffee is actually loaded with antioxidants. Numerous studies show that coffee drinkers live longer and have a lower risk of many serious diseases.

Myth 8: Eating Fat Makes You Fat... So If You Want to Lose Weight, You Need to Eat Less Fat

Fat is the stuff that is under our skin, making us look soft and puffy.

Therefore it seems logical that eating fat would give us even more of it.

However, this depends entirely on the context. Diets that are high in fat AND carbs can make you fat, but it's not because of the fat.

In fact, diets that are high in fat (but low in carbs) consistently lead to more weight loss than low-fat diets... even when the low-fat groups restrict calories (35, 36, 37).

The fattening effects of dietary fat depend entirely on the context. A diet that is high in fat but low in carbs leads to more weight loss than a low-fat diet.

229

Myth 9: A High-Protein Diet Increases Strain on the Kidneys and Raises Your Risk of Kidney Disease

It is often said that dietary protein increases strain on the kidneys and raises the risk of kidney failure.

Although it is true that people with established kidney disease should cut back on protein, this is absolutely not true of otherwise healthy people.

Numerous studies, even in athletes that eat large amounts of protein, show that a high protein intake is perfectly safe

In fact, a higher protein intake lowers blood pressure and helps fight type 2 diabetes... which are two of the main risk factors for kidney failure

Also let's not forget that protein reduces appetite and supports weight loss, but obesity is another strong risk factor for kidney failure

Eating a lot of protein has no adverse effects on kidney function in otherwise healthy people and improves numerous risk factors.

Myth 10: Full-Fat Dairy Products Are High in Saturated Fat and Calories... Raising the Risk of Heart Disease and Obesity

High-fat dairy products are among the richest sources of saturated fat in the diet and very high in calories.

For this reason, we've been told to eat low-fat dairy products instead.

However, the studies do not support this. Eating full-fat dairy product is not linked to increased heart disease and is even associated with a lower risk of obesity.

In countries where cows are grass-fed, eating full-fat dairy is actually associated with up to a 69% lower risk of heart disease

If anything, the main benefits of dairy are due to the fatty components. Therefore, choosing low-fat dairy products is a terrible idea.

Of course... this does not mean that you should go overboard and pour massive amounts of butter in your coffee, but it does imply that reasonable amounts of full-fat dairy from grass-fed cows are both safe and healthy.

Despite being high in saturated fat and calories, studies show that full-fat dairy is linked to a reduced risk of obesity. In countries where cows are grass-fed, full-fat dairy is linked to reduced heart disease.

Myth 11: All Calories Are Created Equal, It Doesn't Matter Which Types of Foods They Are Coming From

It is simply false that "all calories are created equal." Different foods go through different metabolic pathways and have direct effects on fat burning and the hormones and brain centers that regulate appetite

A high protein diet, for example, can increase the metabolic rate by 80 to 100 calories per day and significantly reduce appetite

In one study, such a diet made people automatically eat 441 fewer calories per day. They also lost 11 pounds in 12 weeks, just by adding protein to their diet

There are many more examples of different foods having vastly different effects on hunger, hormones and health. Because a calorie is not a calorie.

Not all calories are created equal, because different foods and macronutrients go through different metabolic pathways. They have varying effects on hunger, hormones and health.

Myth 12: Low-Fat Foods Are Healthy Because They Are Lower in Calories and Saturated Fat

When the low-fat guidelines first came out, the food manufacturers responded with all sorts of low-fat "health foods." The problem is... these foods taste horrible when the fat is removed, so the food manufacturers added a whole bunch of sugar instead.

The truth is, excess sugar is incredibly harmful, while the fat naturally present in food is not.

Processed low-fat foods tend to be very high in sugar, which is very unhealthy compared to the fat that is naturally present in foods.

Myth 13: Red Meat Consumption Raises the Risk of All Sorts of Diseases... Including

Heart Disease, Type 2 Diabetes and Cancer

We are constantly warned about the "dangers" of eating red meat.

It is true that some studies have shown negative effects, but they were usually lumping processed and unprocessed meat together.

The largest studies (one with over 1 million people, the other with over 400 thousand) show that unprocessed red meat is not linked to increased heart disease or type 2 diabetes

Two review studies have also shown that the link to cancer is not as strong as some people would have you believe. The association is weak in men and nonexistent in women

So... don't be afraid of eating meat. Just make sure to eat unprocessed meat and don't overcook it, because eating too much burnt meat may be harmful.

It is a myth that eating unprocessed red meat raises the risk of heart disease and diabetes. The cancer link is also exaggerated, the largest studies find only a weak effect in men and no effect in women.

Myth 14: The Only People Who Should Go Gluten-Free Are Patients With Celiac Disease, About 1% of the Population

It is often claimed that no one benefits from a gluten-free diet except patients with celiac disease. This is the most severe form of gluten intolerance, affecting under 1% of people

But another condition called gluten sensitivity is much more common and may affect about 6-8% of people, although there are no good statistics available yet

Studies have also shown that gluten-free diets can reduce symptoms of irritable bowel syndrome, schizophrenia, autism and epilepsy

However... people should eat foods that are naturally gluten free (like plants and animals), not gluten-free "products." Gluten-free junk food is still junk food.

But keep in mind that the gluten situation is actually quite complicated and there are no clear answers yet. Some new studies suggest that it may be other compounds in wheat that cause some of the digestive problems, not the gluten itself.

Studies have shown that many people can benefit from a gluten-free diet, not just patients with celiac disease.

Myth 15: Losing Weight Is All About Willpower and Eating Less, Exercising More

Weight loss (and gain) is often assumed to be all about willpower and "calories in vs calories out." But this is completely inaccurate.

The human body is a highly complex biological system with many hormones and brain centers that regulate when, what and how much we eat.

It is well known that genetics, hormones and various external factors have a huge impact on body weight

Junk food can also be downright addictive, making people quite literally lose control over their consumption

Although it is still the individual's responsiblity to do something about their weight problem, blaming obesity on some sort of moral failure is unhelpful and inaccurate.

It is a myth that weight gain is caused by some sort of moral failure. Genetics, hormones and all sorts of external factors have a huge effect.

Myth 16: Saturated Fats and Trans Fats Are Similar... They're the "Bad" Fats That We Need to Avoid

The mainstream health organizations often lump saturated and artificial trans fats in the same category... calling them the "bad" fats.

It is true that trans fats are harmful. They are linked to insulin resistance and metabolic problems, drastically raising the risk of heart disease

However, saturated fat is harmless, so it makes absolutely no sense to group the two together.

Interestingly, these same organizations also advise us to eat vegetable oils like soybean and canola oils.

But these oils are actually loaded with unhealthy fats... one study found that 0.56-4.2% of the fatty acids in them are toxic trans fats!

Many mainstream health organizations lump trans fats and saturated fats together, which makes no sense. Trans fats are harmful, saturated fats are not.

Myth 17: Protein Leaches Calcium From the Bones and Raises the Risk of Osteoporosis

It is commonly believed that eating protein raises the acidity of the blood and leaches calcium from the bones, leading to osteoporosis.

Although it is true that a high protein intake increases calcium excretion in the short-term, this effect does not persist in the long-term.

The truth is that a high protein intake is linked to a massively reduced risk of osteoporosis and fractures in old age.

This is one example of where blindly following the conventional nutritional wisdom will have the exact opposite effect of what was intended!

Numerous studies have shown that eating more (not less) protein is linked to a reduced risk of osteoporosis and fractures.

Myth 18: Low-Carb Diets Are Dangerous and Increase Your Risk of Heart Disease

Low-carb diets have been popular for many decades now.

Mainstream nutrition professionals have constantly warned us that these diets will end up clogging our arteries.

However, since the year 2002, over 20 studies have been conducted on the low-carb diet.

Low-carb diets actually cause more weight loss and improve most risk factors for heart disease more than the low-fat diet

Although the tide is slowly turning, many "experts" still claim that such diets are dangerous, then continue to promote the failed low-fat dogma that science has shown to be utterly useless.

Of course, low-carb diets are not for everyone, but it is very clear that they can have major benefits for people with obesity, type 2 diabetes and metabolic syndrome... some of the biggest health problems in the world

Despite having been demonized in the past, many new studies have shown that low-carb diets are much healthier than the low-fat diet still recommended by the mainstream.

Myth 19: Sugar Is Mainly Harmful Because of It Supplies "Empty" Calories"

Pretty much everyone agrees that sugar is unhealthy when consumed in excess.

But many people still believe that it is only bad because it supplies empty calories.

Well... nothing could be farther from the truth.

When consumed in excess, sugar can cause severe metabolic problems

Many experts now believe that sugar may be driving of some of the world's biggest killers... including obesity, heart disease, diabetes and even cancer

Although sugar is fine in small amounts (especially for those who are physically active and metabolically healthy), it can be a complete disaster when consumed in excess.

Myth 20: Refined Seed and Vegetable Oils Like Soybean and Corn Oils Lower Cholesterol and Are Super Healthy

Vegetable oils like soybean and corn oils are high in Omega-6 polyunsaturated fats, which have been shown to lower cholesterol levels.

But it's important to remember that cholesterol is a risk factor for heart disease, not a disease in itself.

Just because something improves a risk factor, it doesn't mean that it will affect hard end points like heart attacks or death... which is what really counts.

The truth is that several studies have shown that these oils increase the risk of death, from both heart disease and cancer

Even though these oils have been shown to cause heart disease and kill people, the mainstream health organizations are still telling us to eat them.

BIGGEST MISTAKES YOU'RE MAKING ON AN ANTI-INFLAMMATORY DIET

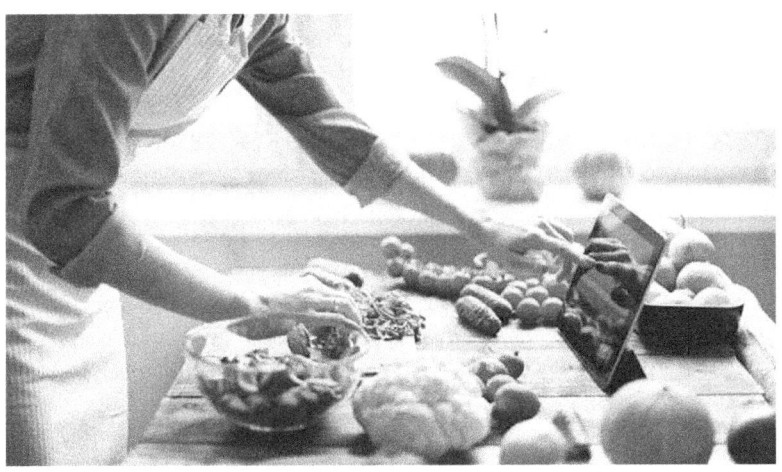

REDUCING CHRONIC INFLAMMATION in the body by way of eating delicious, nutrient-dense foods sound like a dream, but the benefits are as real as it gets.

Inflammation is a healthy response by your immune system that helps your body heal from injury and fights off pathogens like viruses and bacteria. Inflammation becomes harmful when your immune system is triggered into a state of chronic inflammation that runs rampant in your body. In fact, chronic inflammation is at the root of most chronic health conditions and, food is one of the most common triggers of inflammation.

As a nutritionist with an anti-inflammatory approach, I work with clients to help them reduce chronic inflammation in the body. If you're wondering what inflammation is and why you might want to try an anti-inflammatory diet, here is some helpful information.

Is There A Food-Inflammation Connection?

To understand the food-inflammation connection, we look to the gut which has proteins called tight junctions that bind the cells of your gut wall together so that food particles and other substances don't leak through. When you eat food that damages your gut lining, those tight junctions open and enable food particles and other substances to leak through, causing intestinal permeability or leaky gut. This is a problem because the immune cells located just beneath your gut wall identify the food particles as harmful foreign invaders and begin reacting to them. As a consequence, you're left with chronic inflammation, food sensitivities and many resulting symptoms.

Food sensitivity symptoms can manifest anywhere from hours to days after you eat a problem food and can include: skin rashes, acne, excess sweating, hives, fatigue, headaches, migraines, gastrointestinal symptoms, mood issues, asthma, weight management issues, bloating, water retention, muscle pain, joint pain, sinus problems and runny nose, among others.

What Are Considered Anti-Inflammatory Foods?

The best way to combat food-induced inflammation is by adopting an anti-inflammatory diet. On an anti-inflammatory diet, you eat real, whole foods and incorporate anti-inflammatory foods, including:

ginger

turmeric

rosemary

wild Alaskan salmon

oregano

green tea

berries

cacao

cinnamon

garlic

extra-virgin olive oil

flax seeds

tart cherry juice

walnuts

olives

vegetables

Now Tell Me About The Elimination Diet...

When starting an anti-inflammatory diet, an elimination diet is considered the gold standard for helping figure out which foods are inflammatory for your particular system. During an elimination diet, you remove foods that are common inflammatory triggers for a large percentage of the population, such as:

gluten

dairy

soy

corn

eggs

sugar

refined vegetable oils

trans fats

artificial foods

processed foods

fried foods

foods cooked at high heat

refined carbs

Then, after eliminating these foods for a set period of time, you begin to reintroduce some of them one by one to test which may be causing food sensitivity symptoms (see below for more specifics). Keep in mind that if you reduce inflammation and support your gut, in three to six months you can retest a food that you initially reacted to. You may find you do not have any symptoms.

How Do I Start The Anti-Inflammatory Diet?

If you're feeling inspired to eat this way, it's important to set yourself up for success. Even if you understand the basics of the anti-inflammatory diet, it's easy to get tripped up when you're trying it in real life. You should feel empowered to successfully implement the anti-inflammatory diet in your life and stick with it long term.

Here are the most common mistakes that people make when starting an anti-inflammatory diet and how to avoid them:

USING THE ELIMINATION DIET PERMANENTLY Sometimes people feel so amazing during an elimination diet they want to skip the testing component and just stay on the elimination diet forever. But the purpose of an elimination diet is to temporarily restrict certain foods so you can identify which of those foods are inflammatory — it's not to permanently restrict healthy foods from your diet that aren't causing food sensitivity symptoms. People also often remain on an elimination diet indefinitely because they don't know what to reintroduce and so they don't test anything at all. To help you figure out what to test and what not to, here's the cheat sheet:

- There are plenty of nutrient-rich foods that you remove on an elimination diet such as eggs, bell peppers, eggplant and tomatoes — but these foods are a great addition to your diet if they don't cause food sensitivity symptoms. Test these foods.

- Foods with no nutritional value like artificial foods, processed foods and refined carbs are best left out of your diet. You don't need to test these foods.

- Although whole food-based, leave gluten-containing grains out of your diet, even if you don't experience food sensitivity symptoms when you eat them. The reason is that gluten can trigger the release of zonulin, a protein that opens up those tight junctions that bind the cells in the lining of your gut, causing leaky gut.

- Most people feel better leaving dairy out of their diet. However, if you'd like to try adding dairy back in, test it. If you're able to consume dairy without experiencing any symptoms, eat it sparingly and make sure that you choose organic, grass-fed sources that are ethically and humanely produced.

You can also try testing soy and corn, but keep this in mind:

- Make sure you choose organic to avoid exposure to genetically modified sources, which have been engineered to be resistant to the highly toxic herbicide glyphosate.

- If you're going to eat soy, choose fermented sources (like natto and tempeh) and steer clear of the processed versions found in packaged foods.

EATING ORGANIC, GLUTEN-FREE, VEGAN-REFINED CARBS When you start an anti-inflammatory diet and look for swaps for the foods you used to eat, it might be tempting to eat lots of organic, gluten-free and vegan refined carbs such as cookies, chips, pretzels and crackers. But labels like "organic" "gluten-free" and "vegan" don't make any food inherently healthy, and foods with these labels can still be and often are inflammatory.

For example, an organic, gluten-free vegan hot dog bun made from refined flour is totally devoid of nutrients and will still trigger inflammation and spike your blood sugar, even if it's organic and made without gluten or dairy. So, when making substitutions, avoid refined carbs and instead aim to choose swaps made from whole food ingredients.

ADOPTING A DIET MENTALITY | If you only plan to stay on an anti-inflammatory diet until you reach a particular goal, like losing five pounds for example, and then revert to how you ate before, you are defeating the whole purpose of eating this way. Ditch the diet mentality and instead look at this anti-inflammatory nutritional approach as one of the most important lifestyle changes you'll ever make to elevate your health long term. Then, to enable yourself to actually stick with it, focus on finding healthy, delicious ingredient and recipe replacements to take the place of the inflammatory foods you used to eat.

NOT HONORING YOU | Don't let overwhelm prevent you from changing your diet. If it feels too daunting to fully adopt an anti-inflammatory diet right now, ask yourself what would be feasible and start there. In other words, pick one change you feel you're ready to make and commit to integrating it in your life. Once it feels sustainable and effortless — whether it's one day, week or month from now — pick another. Then another. Then another. Before you know it, you will have totally transformed the way you eat, and you will have done it at a pace that was right for you.

BELIEVING ANTI-INFLAMMATORY FOODS CANCEL OUT INFLAMMATORY FOODS | Take as much time as you need to transition to an anti-inflammatory diet while keeping in mind that anti-inflammatory foods can't cancel the impact that inflammatory foods have on your body. So, if you're still eating cheeseburgers and French fries for lunch and dinner, that fish oil supplement and sprinkle of flax seeds on your breakfast while a great start won't help you escape food-induced inflammation.

WHOLE30 DIET FOODS

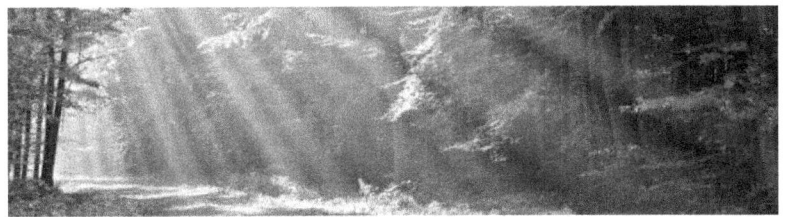

Can Whole30 change your life? We asked an expert to weigh in on this popular eating plan.

Our highly-processed, modern diets trigger inflammation, hormone imbalances, and subtle food intolerances in the body, and the combined effect has a cascading effect on our health, appetite, and cravings. This is the premise behind Whole30, a food "reset" centered around eating only whole, unprocessed or very minimally processed foods.

Struggling to cook healthy? We'll help you prep.

Sign up for our new weekly newsletter, ThePrep, for inspiration and support for all your meal plan struggles.

Focusing on healthy eating changes albeit pretty drastic for most people for a set time period is much more appealing when compared to diets with an infinite end. But how much impact can the Whole30 program really have on health, food cravings, and future food choices? Better yet, is it a safe way to eat long-term? Here's everything you need to know.

What Is Whole30?

By following Whole30 guidelines which include cutting out foods triggering inflammation and imbalances for 30 days you can effectively "calm" your body down. After eating "clean" for 30 days, you can continue with the program or slowly add restricted foods back into your diet. This way, you'll be able to effectively identify which ones may be having subtle effects on your health.

Meals during the 30 day-period center around lots of vegetables, moderate amounts of protein from meat, poultry, seafood, and eggs, some fruits, and healthy fats from foods like nuts, seeds, oils, avocados and olives. Nut milks and nut butters are allowed, as well as all spices and herbs.

Now, here's what you must eliminate or avoid:

All added sugars and artificial sweeteners

Grains (refined and whole)

Legumes, peas, and soy products

Dairy

Highly processed foods and foods with certain additives

Alcohol

While Whole30 isn't usually marketed as low-carb, eating on this plan tends to be lower in carbohydrates. And because some fruits and starchy vegetables like sweet potatoes are encouraged, Whole30 isn't nearly as carb-scarce as the Atkins diet or Keto diet.

In fact, from a macronutrient prospective, a day of Whole30 eating isn't too far off from the current health recommendations (45-65% carbs, 20-35% fat, and 15-25% protein). Here's how a typical Whole30 day breaks down: approximately 35-50% from calories from carbs, 25-35% from fat calories, and 25-35% from protein calories.

What's the Difference Between Whole30 and Paleo?

Whole30 and the Paleo diet both surged in popularity a few years ago around the same time (when their respective books hit the market), and they have lots of similarities. Both diets focus on eating whole, unprocessed foods and cutting out added sugars, grains, legumes, dairy, and processed foods.

However, there are several key differences between the two diets. Whole30 is a strict, 30-day reset period that some then choose to adopt as a long-term eating approach. The Paleo diet, on the other hand, is viewed as a long-term way of living and eating that emphasizes grass-fed, sustainable proteins and local produce. Lastly, nutrient intakes of Paleo followers tend to be a little higher in protein and saturated fat.

Potential Health Benefits of Whole30

While eating according to the Whole30 guidelines may initiate some of these health improvements, this isn't the full picture. These changes aren't necessarily triggered by Whole30 itself but rather the act of following an elimination diet that emphasizes anti-inflammatory eating.

Elimination diets are therapeutic eating protocols that health practitioners have used for years. When a person is plagued by vague, but ongoing symptoms like digestive issues, headaches, joint pain, or skin conditions, they are especially useful in identifying food sensitivities. However, unlike food allergies, food sensitivities are difficult to detect through testing.

Continued consumption of trigger foods can contribute to low-level inflammation and imbalances in the body. Now combines an unknown potential food sensitivity with the typical American diet high in foods that trigger chronic inflammation—added sugars, fried foods, refined carbs, artificial sweeteners, excess alcohol, processed meats, and saturated and trans fats—and you've got a perpetual cycle of inflammation. Research has demonstrated that this type of inflammation increases risks for cancer, type 2 diabetes, heart disease, metabolic syndrome, some autoimmune diseases, and possibly brain alterations.

This is a modal window.

Whole30 is essentially a consumer-friendly version of an elimination diet that cuts out potential food sensitivities for 30 days, as well as drastically decreases inflammatory food intake and increases key anti-inflammatory foods like fruits, vegetables, and omega-3 fatty acids. Whether you have an unidentified food sensitivity or not, the overall effect of eating like this eases inflammation so you could see subtle health improvements related to digestion, skin, headaches, and joint pain.

Potential Problems with Whole30

While the Whole30 diet may be a good "kick-off" for an anti-inflammatory or clean eating approach, its guidelines don't align with research and health recommendations. Among the biggest concerns are the restrictiveness and avoidance of certain food groups. Here are four problems health professionals have when considering this diet as a long-term eating plan:

1. Elimination diets are meant to be temporary.

While extremely helpful to identify foods triggering issues, elimination diets are also very restrictive. They're designed to be a temporary diagnosis tool—and not a permanent way of eating. Elimination diets recommend avoiding certain foods for 4 to 6 weeks, then slowly adding them back one-by-one to identify any triggering issues.

Because Whole30 guidelines don't require the re-entry of restricted foods after 30 days, you may be putting yourself at risk for nutrient deficiencies. Calcium and Vitamin D deficiencies are the biggest concerns, but magnesium, folate, Vitamin A, Vitamin E and others may be affected if you aren't getting an adequate variety of produce and healthy fats.

2. Avoiding Whole Grains.

Consuming whole grains is associated with lowering inflammatory markers in the body and has demonstrated a protective effect when it comes to diabetes and heart disease. The Mediterranean Diet is a key model for anti-inflammatory eating and suggests whole grains be a staple part of one's diet. And unless you're sensitive or allergic to gluten or specific grain, research only supports avoiding refined grains.

3. Avoiding Legumes.

Paleo and Whole30 diets are largely responsible for planting the seeds that beans and legumes should be avoided due to their anti-nutrients. However, these compounds typically have little negative effect on the body—or not nearly enough to outweigh the benefits—when beans are consumed a few times per week. The Mediterranean Diet also recommends legumes as a key source of protein and high-fiber, low-glycemic carbs.

4. Avoiding Dairy.

Unless you have a dairy allergy or sensitivity, there's little research to support avoiding dairy long-term. In fact, dairy products have an anti-inflammatory effect in most people, especially yogurt.

What's the Verdict on Whole30?

The Whole30 diet is a quick snapshot of a healthy, but pretty restrictive, eating pattern. If you frequently consume highly-processed foods and are looking to adopt a healthier lifestyle, you may find the strict parameters helpful. However, research suggests that healthy eating doesn't has to be nearly as limited as the Whole30 guidelines.

ANTI-INFLAMMATORY DIET LIFESTYLE GUIDE

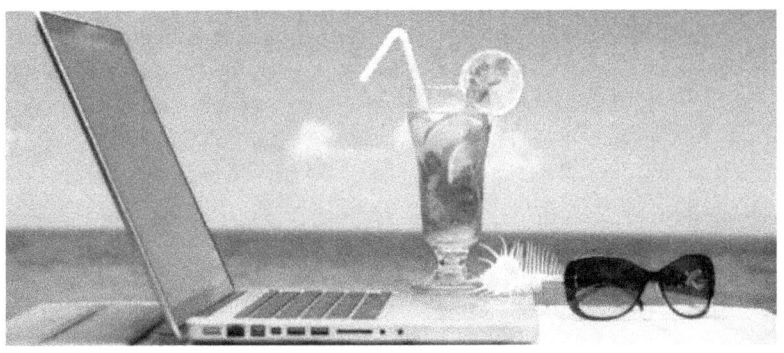

No one among us is utterly immune to inflammation. Even the healthiest people are tripped up at times by a cut on their finger or waylaid by a common cold or flu. Unfortunately, for many of us inflammation is a constant, chronic problem – aches and pains, allergies, autoimmune conditions, cardiovascular disease, diabetes, respiratory issues and more all involve inflammation; it affects millions of people around the world and costs us billions of dollars. The good news is an anti-inflammatory diet and lifestyle can play an important role in the prevention and management of inflammatory symptoms. And it can be delicious!

If you're interested in learning more about how an anti-inflammatory diet can help you, we're sharing our Anti-Inflammatory Diet Guide today. Whether you or someone you love is dealing with inflammation, we hope that you can discover some new ways to address it using our tips and advice.

Dietary changes take time and effort; so don't feel pressured to do everything at once. Incorporate one thing at a time at a pace that feels right to you!

1. Eliminate Sources of Gluten

Gluten, which is found in wheat, barley and rye, is linked to inflammation and can affect the intestinal wall – particles can break through into the bloodstream where they don't belong, leading to an immune response. Gluten has become quite a controversial topic in recent years, with many experts claiming that only those with celiac disease benefit from avoiding and eliminating gluten. However, there are many inflammatory conditions that can benefit from a gluten-free diet, especially those that are autoimmune.

There is no nutrient found in glutenous products that we can't find elsewhere in the diet and in many cases, ditching gluten involves cutting out the junk food like white bread, pizza, pastries, etc. We recommend trying a gluten-free diet for at least two weeks to see how you feel, then adjust accordingly.

2. Ditch the Dairy

Dairy products, especially those made from cow's milk, can be difficult to digest. Many of us don't produce the lactase enzyme required to process the lactose in milk, which can lead to poor digestion and bloating, gas or cramps. Some people react to the proteins in milk like whey and casein and casein is actually similar in structure to gluten.

3. Avoid White, Refined Sugar

It's probably not breaking news to you that refined sugars are damaging to our health. Excess sugar and refined starches spike insulin levels, can boost our body's production of inflammatory chemicals, not to mention that sugar is linked to obesity, diabetes, tooth decay and mood swings.

Thankfully, there are many natural sweeteners available like dates, raw honey, coconut sugar, coconut syrup, maple syrup, etc. And let's not forget about the natural sugars found in fruit, which can be the best dessert of all.

4. Mind The Nightshade Family

The nightshade family includes tomatoes, eggplant, peppers, white potatoes, goji berries and tobacco. Some people are sensitive to nightshade plants, particularly one phytochemical called solanine. Nightshades can impact inflammation, particularly arthritis.

Nightshades can be a tricky food category to navigate, since they also have a multitude of beneficial properties. If you're dealing with inflammation, try cutting them out for a month and see if it makes a difference. You can also rotate nightshades in your diet, as opposed to having them on a daily or weekly basis.

5. Load up on Anti-Inflammatory Foods

The good news is there are a ton – a ton – of delicious anti-inflammatory foods you can include in your diet. These foods are simple to use and easy to find at most grocery stores or farmers markets.

Dark Leafy Greens. These are packed with anti-oxidants that help to ameliorate the effects of inflammation. They also contain a wide variety of other beneficial vitamins and minerals, including B vitamins, iron, magnesium and calcium.

Winter Squash. Winter squash contains curcubitacins, which halt the production of enzymes that lead to inflammation, and they are loaded with immune-supportive Vitamins A and C. Learn more about how awesome they are in this Guide to Winter Squash.

Cruciferous Vegetables. Broccoli, kale, Brussels sprouts, cabbage and cauliflower all help to reduce inflammation and they are a fantastic culinary family to use when detoxing.

Allium Family. Grab onions, garlic, leeks, shallots or chives the next time you're at the grocery store. They contain sulfur compounds and other molecules that avert inflammation; they are also a source of Vitamin C and can help boost the immune system.

Berries. These heavenly fruits are high in a wide range of anti-inflammatory antioxidants.

Fish. Fish is an incredible source of omega-3 fatty acids, which are highly anti-inflammatory, and it's high in protein – an essential macronutrient for healing and repair.

Nuts and Seeds. These are wonderful plant-based option for omega-3s (especially hemp seeds, flax seeds, chia seeds and walnuts). They are also protein-rich and high in fibre.

6. Experiment with Herbs + Spices

There are a range of potent herbs and spices you can add to your pantry that prevent and reduce inflammation, plus they add extra flavour to your meals. Some amazing ones to start off with are ginger, turmeric, fennel, parsley and cumin – but experiment away and see which ones you love to use.

7. Drink Water – And Lots of It

Hydration supports the digestive system, the urinary tract, our joints and our skin; water even helps with energy levels and weight loss. Skip bottled water, which is stored in plastic and is often just tap water. Instead, source the cleanest water you can find, whether that's through buying a water filter or collecting it from a local spring. There are plenty of options out there, and the filters you buy will depend on where you live and what's in your water.

And if you're sick of drinking water plain, here are a few infused water options to jazz things up.

8. Move Your Body

Research indicates that exercise can stimulate anti-inflammatory chemicals in the body and reduce inflammation. Even 20 minutes of exercise like walking is beneficial, so you don't need to run triathlons to reap the benefits. If you're in a lot of pain or are in the midst of a flare up, aim for gentle exercise like walking, swimming, rebounding, hatha or yin yoga, or anything you enjoy at a lighter or more relaxed pace.

9. Lower Stress Levels

Psychological stress can dampen our ability to fight and regulate inflammation. Aim to lower and reduce your stress levels as much as possible; whether it's through yoga and meditation, being out in nature, or eating stress-busting foods, find your stress-reducing sweet spot and live there as much as possible!

It is becoming increasingly clear that chronic inflammation is the root cause of many serious illnesses including heart disease, many cancers, and Alzheimer's disease. We all know inflammation on the surface of the body as local redness, heat, swelling and pain. It is the cornerstone of the body's healing response, bringing more nourishment and more immune activity to a site of injury or infection. But when inflammation persists or serves no purpose, it damages the body and causes illness. Stress, lack of exercise, genetic predisposition, and exposure to toxins (like secondhand tobacco smoke) can all contribute to such chronic inflammation, but dietary choices play a big role as well. Learning how specific foods influence the inflammatory process is the best strategy for containing it and reducing long-term disease risks.

The Anti Inflammatory Food Pyramid Now!

The Anti-Inflammatory Diet is not a diet in the popular sense – it is not intended as a weight-loss program (although people can and do lose weight on it), nor is the Anti-Inflammatory Diet an eating plan to stay on for a limited period of time. Rather, it is way of selecting and preparing anti-inflammatory foods based on scientific knowledge of

255

how they can help your body maintain optimum health. Along with influencing inflammation, this natural anti-inflammatory diet will provide steady energy and ample vitamins, minerals, essential fatty acids dietary fiber, and protective phytonutrients.

General Anti-Inflammatory Diet Tips:

Aim for variety.

Include as much fresh food as possible.

Minimize your consumption of processed foods and fast food.

Eat an abundance of fruits and vegetables.

Caloric Intake

Most adults need to consume between 2,000 and 3,000 calories a day.

Women and smaller and less active people need fewer calories.

Men and bigger and more active people need more calories.

If you are eating the appropriate number of calories for your level of activity, your weight should not fluctuate greatly.

The distribution of calories you take in should be as follows: 40 to 50 percent from carbohydrates, 30 percent from fat, and 20 to 30 percent from protein.

Try to include carbohydrates, fat, and protein at each meal.

Carbohydrates

On a 2,000-calorie-a-day diet, adult women should consume between 160 to 200 grams of carbohydrates a day.

Adult men should consume between 240 to 300 grams of carbohydrates a day.

The majority of this should be in the form of less-refined, less-processed foods with a low glycemic load.

Reduce your consumption of foods made with wheat flour and sugar, especially bread and most packaged snack foods (including chips and pretzels).

Eat more whole grains such as brown rice and bulgur wheat, in which the grain is intact or in a few large pieces. These are preferable to whole wheat flour products, which have roughly the same glycemic index as white flour products.

Eat more beans, winter squashes, and sweet potatoes.

Cook pasta al dente and eat it in moderation.

Avoid products made with high fructose corn syrup.

Fat

On a 2,000-calorie-a-day diet, 600 calories can come from fat – that is, about 67 grams. This should be in a ratio of 1:2:1 of saturated to monounsaturated to polyunsaturated fat.

Reduce your intake of saturated fat by eating less butter, cream, high-fat cheese, unskinned chicken and fatty meats, and products made with palm kernel oil.

Use extra-virgin olive oil as a main cooking oil. If you want a neutral tasting oil, use expeller-pressed, organic canola oil. Organic, high-oleic, expeller pressed versions of sunflower and safflower oil are also acceptable.

Avoid regular safflower and sunflower oils, corn oil, cottonseed oil, and mixed vegetable

oils.

Strictly avoid margarine, vegetable shortening, and all products listing them as ingredients. Strictly avoid all products made with partially hydrogenated oils of any kind. Include in your diet avocados and nuts, especially walnuts, cashews, almonds, and nut butters made from these nuts.

For omega-3 fatty acids, eat salmon (preferably fresh or frozen wild or canned sockeye), sardines packed in water or olive oil, herring, and black cod (sablefish, butterfish); omega-3 fortified eggs; hemp seeds and flaxseeds (preferably freshly ground); or take a fish oil supplement (look for products that provide both EPA and DHA, in a convenient daily dosage of two to three grams).

Protein

On a 2,000-calorie-a-day diet, your daily intake of protein should be between 80 and 120 grams. Eat less protein if you have liver or kidney problems, allergies, or autoimmune disease.

Decrease your consumption of animal protein except for fish and high quality natural cheese and yogurt.

Eat more vegetable protein, especially from beans in general and soybeans in particular. Become familiar with the range of whole-soy foods available and find ones you like.

Fiber

Try to eat 40 grams of fiber a day. You can achieve this by increasing your consumption of fruit, especially berries, vegetables (especially beans), and whole grains.

Ready-made cereals can be good fiber sources, but read labels to make sure they give you at least 4 and preferably 5 grams of bran per one-ounce serving.

Phytonutrients

To get maximum natural protection against age-related diseases (including cardiovascular disease, cancer, and neurodegenerative disease) as well as against environmental toxicity, eat a variety of fruits, vegetables and mushrooms.

Choose fruits and vegetables from all parts of the color spectrum, especially berries, tomatoes, orange and yellow fruits, and dark leafy greens.

Choose organic produce whenever possible. Learn which conventionally grown crops are most likely to carry pesticide residues and avoid them.

Eat cruciferous (cabbage-family) vegetables regularly.

Include soy foods in your diet.

Drink tea instead of coffee, especially good quality white, green or oolong tea.

If you drink alcohol, use red wine preferentially.

Enjoy plain dark chocolate in moderation (with a minimum cocoa content of 70 percent).

Vitamins and Minerals

The best way to obtain all of your daily vitamins, minerals, and micronutrients is by eating a diet high in fresh foods with an abundance of fruits and vegetables. In addition, supplement your diet with the following antioxidant cocktail:

Vitamin C, 200 milligrams a day.

Vitamin E. Most adults should limit their daily supplement intake of vitamin E to 100-200 IU (in the form of mixed tocopherols and tocotrienols).

Selenium, 100-200 micrograms per day.

Mixed carotenoids, 10,000-15,000 IU daily.

The antioxidants can be most conveniently taken as part of a daily multivitamin/multimineral supplement. It should contain no iron (unless you are a female and having regular menstrual periods) and no preformed vitamin A (retinol). Take these supplements with your largest meal.

Women should take supplemental calcium, preferably as calcium citrate, 500-700 milligrams a day, depending on their dietary intake of this mineral. Men should avoid supplemental calcium.

Other Measures To Consider

If you are not eating oily fish at least twice a week, take supplemental fish oil, in capsule or liquid form (two to three grams a day of a product containing both EPA and DHA). Look for molecularly distilled products certified to be free of heavy metals and other contaminants.

Talk to your doctor about going on low-dose aspirin therapy, one or two baby aspirins a day (81 or 162 milligrams).

If you are not regularly eating ginger and turmeric, consider taking these in supplemental form.

Add coenzyme Q10 (CoQ10) to your daily regimen: 60-100 milligrams of a softgel form taken with your largest meal.

If you are prone to metabolic syndrome, take alpha-lipoic acid, 100 to 400 milligrams a day.

Water

Drink pure water, or drinks that are mostly water (tea, very diluted fruit juice, sparkling water with lemon) throughout the day.

Use bottled water or get a home water purifier if your tap water tastes of chlorine or other contaminants, or if you live in an area where the water is known or suspected to be contaminated.